Accident and Emerg

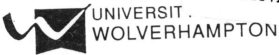

UNIVERSIT
WOLVERHAMPTON

Harrison Learning Centre
Wolverhampton Campus
University of Wolverhampton
St Peter's Square
Wolverhampton WV1 1RH
Telephone: 0845 408 1?2

)0

Accident and Emergency Nursing

A nursing model

Lynn Sbaih

Lecturer to the Accident and Emergency
Nursing Course, Stoke-on-Trent

CHAPMAN & HALL

London · Glasgow · New York · Tokyo · Melbourne · Madras

Published by Chapman & Hall, 2–6 Boundary Row, London SE1 8HN

Chapman & Hall, 2–6 Boundary Row, London SE1 8HN, UK

Blackie Academic & Professional, Wester Cleddens Road,
Bishopbriggs, Glasgow G64 2NZ, UK

Chapman & Hall, 29 West 35th Street, New York NY10001, USA

Chapman & Hall Japan, Thomson Publishing Japan,
Hirakawacho Nemoto Building, 7F,
1–7–11 Hirakawa–cho, Chiyoda–ku, Tokyo 102, Japan

Chapman & Hall Australia, Thomas Nelson Australia,
102 Dodds Street, South Melbourne, Victoria 3205, Australia

Chapman & Hall India, R. Seshadri,
32 Second Main Road, CIT East, Madras 600 035, India

Distributed in the USA and Canada by Singular Publishing Group,
Inc., 4284 41st Street, San Diego, California 92105

First edition 1992

© 1992 Chapman & Hall

Typeset in 10½ on 12pt Palatino by Falcon Typographic Art Ltd,
Fife, Scotland
Printed in Great Britain at the University Press, Cambridge

ISBN 0 412 41180 6   1 56593 031 2 (USA)

A catalogue record for this book is available from the British Library

For Eyad

'The shortest answer is doing'

Lord Herbert
(1583–1648)
English philosopher and diplomat

Contents

Acknowledgements

This book grew out of a number of suggestions made in relation to the practical use of a nursing model. For this I thank Phil.

The suggestions led to ideas, and those ideas to more ideas. Eventually a document based upon a nursing model evolved. My thanks to all the staff in the A and E department at the Northern General Hospital, Sheffield for making this possible. Also, my thanks to Karen for continuing to monitor and develop the work there.

My thanks to my friends and colleagues for their support, advice and encouragement. In particular to Lynne, Freya and Janet for listening to my numerous ideas as the book developed.

Thank you to Steve Wright for his help and suggestion that I write this book. Also, to Rosemary who has always been available for discussion and advice, and who has encouraged me and has always said the right thing.

Thank you to Betty Kershaw for her support and advice during the final stages of the book.

Finally, my sincere thanks to those not mentioned but by no means forgotten.

Foreword

The majority of people who are admitted to hospital are anxious, even when they are well prepared for admission and confident about the explanations they receive giving details about their stay in hospital. It is not surprising, therefore, that patients admitted to an accident and emergency (A and E) department may also be anxious as they have none of the security of prepared admission. They, their relatives and friends will experience the trauma of physiological pain and shock, of psychological stress and of social anxiety.

There are many different reactions to this trauma, and these will put various demands on nursing staff and the other members of the health care team. Some individuals withdraw, sitting or lying very quietly. Communication is difficult, and there is a danger that these patients can be overlooked merely because they are quiet. There is no chance of overlooking those whose anxiety manifests itself in aggressive or demanding, perhaps even violent, behaviours. This may take the form of constant questioning, or following staff around the department. However, at its worst, and aggravated by alcohol, verbal and physical abuse can follow.

These problems can be aggravated by lengthy delays in receiving attention and treatment. Also, the obvious signs of distress which are shown by other patients can increase the anxiety felt by those who join a seemingly endless queue for care and treatment. Patients who do not have to queue, or who are brought in by ambulance as an emergency, often experience extreme fear and feelings of isolation. This is also true for the person who is left waiting outside a cubicle while urgent treatment is given to someone for whom they care. These feelings often have to be experienced to be believed.

Nowhere is the role of the nurse more important; nowhere is it more vital that the caring intervention offered is of the very best, supported by a high level of knowledge and technical skill, than in areas such as A and E nursing.

Lynn Sbaih is an experienced A and E nurse who now works as a nurse teacher. She is responsible for the ENB 199 A and E nursing course and is involved in teaching pre-registration students, as well as working with one of the busiest trauma units in the country. She has used her undoubted expertise in writing this book which explores, for the first time, the interesting and important application of nursing models to A and E nursing care. Even more important, she has used documented care plans, including the assessment and evaluation of care given. The assessment is, of course, unique to casualty units, in that it recognizes the role of the nurse in triage.

The book is especially of value now as the whole issue of expanded and extended nursing roles is under debate, and as nurses are recognizing their professional autonomy and accountability. Specialist practitioners are developing; we have new roles to explore and new challenges to face.

Lynn is to be congratulated on producing a text which should be of interest both to qualified staff for whom trauma nursing is a career decision as well as to those many more who are interested in how patients are admitted, cared for and discharged from the A and E department of the general hospitals.

Betty Kershaw

Chapter 1

Organization of the A and E department

CONTENTS

- Introduction
- Professions
- Organizational theory
- References

INTRODUCTION

This book addresses the assessment, action and evaluation of care in A and E nursing. Although this is the main aim, a wider range of issues – nursing philosophies, the change process and the implementation of change – will be considered. Much has been written about the adoption and use of nursing models in clinical practice (Fitzpatrick and Whall, 1983; Roper, Logan and Tierney, 1983; Salvage and Kershaw, 1990; Wright, 1986), and nurses' thoughts about the utilization of nursing models will also be discussed. There have been a variety of broad but related themes introduced into the debate about the appropriateness of a nursing model in A and E. These will be discussed as well as specific ideas and information which can then be evaluated by the reader.

The format of the book is such that the use of 'she' will be used, unless specific individuals are described. This is to avoid grammatical clumsiness only, and not intended to ignore the increasing numbers and importance of male nurses entering the profession. In each chapter several themes will be introduced through the presentation of definitions and descriptions from a variety of sources. The reader is invited to consider established facts and, through discussion points, apply these to A and E nursing. Those with a unique knowledge of A and E nursing will be invaluable participants in the discussion. Through previous knowledge and experience of A and E nursing, together with information introduced in each chapter, nurses should be able to analyze and examine specific problems encountered whilst functioning in a variety of roles in the clinical area. Some of the problems considered may relate to the use of a nursing model.

It is not always possible to find solutions to identified problems. However, it is important, through thought and discussion, to continue to explore the issues involved.

In this chapter, theories and definitions related to professions and to the concept of organization will be discussed. These will be examined within the context of A and E nursing. After this, different interpretations of philosophy will be analyzed and disseminated, through the use of discussion points (Chapter 2). Chapter 3 offers a philosophical framework for care, and discusses the implications for practice. This is followed by definitions of the nursing process and nursing models which will be explored and compared. Methods of documentation will also be examined (Chapter 4). Preparation for change, the change process, implementing change and a plan of change will be discussed in chapters 5 and 6. A variety of themes that may affect nurses' reactions, both positive and negative, to the use of nursing models in A and E departments will be examined. Issues, such as stress, role and job satisfaction, will be explored in this context (Chapter 7). Finally, all the themes discussed in the previous chapters will be reintroduced in the last chapter (Chapter 8), and there will be a concluding discussion.

PROFESSIONS

Until recently, sociologists viewed professional persons as 'honoured servants of public need', distinguished from others by 'esoteric knowledge and complex skill' (Friedson, 1983). According to this definition a member of a profession can be defined as a person who provides a service to meet the needs of the public; a person who has a range of skills and knowledge to which the ordinary person has no access.

There have been many other views of professions, and exploration of their organization and place in society (Carr-Saunders, 1928). Some economists, for example, have remarked on the controlling characteristics of professions and their effect on the labour market (Caplow, 1954). Political scientists have described a profession as a 'privileged private government' (Friedson, 1983), and some policy makers believe that professions have limited knowledge and beliefs about 'what is good for the public' (Laski, 1931). These are just a few of the definitions that have been given in the past.

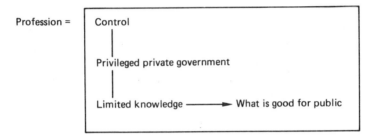

Such views of the professions suggest that the possession of a unique quality divides a profession from other occupations. The distinction between this quality and others is under continual debate (Dingwell, 1976; Friedson, 1970; Illich, 1977).

Points for discussion:

• Which occupations should be referred to as professions?
• What specific qualities, if any, do such occupations possess?

Friedson (1983) offers a variety of definitions including the suggestion that a profession may be 'a changing historical concept with roots in an industrial nation influenced by Anglo-American institutions'. This suggests that many modern professions originate from industrial sources both in Britain and America. Prior to the industrial revolution those occupations viewed as professions today either did not exist or existed in an alternative way.

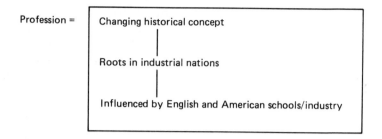

Profession =

| Changing historical concept |
| Roots in industrial nations |
| Influenced by English and American schools/industry |

Points for discussion:

- With reference to this definition discuss the growth of nursing.

Historically, in Europe there have been three professions: medicine, law and the clergy (Elliot, 1972). Recently, however, middle class occupations, in England, have sought the protection of professional status in an attempt to gain respectability (Larson, 1977).

Usage of word profession

1. Collection of individuals

Higher education

Distinctive occupation

Identified by educational status

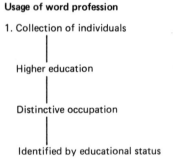

2. Occupation

Intellectual

Conceptual

Traits ⟶ Common

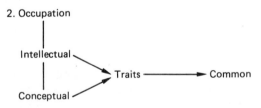

Friedson (1983) continued his discussion by stating that there are two broad definitions of the word profession:

- A collection of individuals identified by their educational status. They will have received higher education and now have distinctive occupations. Specific occupational skills held by them do not necessarily identify them with others;
- A limited number of occupations with specific intellectual and conceptual traits in common.

Johnson (1972) defined professionalism in terms of intellectual and conceptual characteristics, such as those used by Friedson (1983) in his second definition. However, professionalization, according to Vollmer and Mills (1966), is an occupation's move towards a professional model.

Another definition of the professions has evolved from these concepts: 'a fairly limited number of occupations which share characteristics of considerably greater specificity than higher education alone, and which are distinctive as separate occupations. Their members conceive of themselves by their occupation first and by their 'class', if at all, only second' (Friedson, 1983).

The professions

Small number of occupations

|

Share specific characteristics

|

Also function as separate occupations

|

Members identify themselves primarily by occupation

McCormack (1979), when writing about the medical profession, stated that 'professions are distinguished from trades by the length of training, the depth of special knowledge and by codes of behaviour'.

Professional model

Hall (1968) speaks of a professional model (Figure 1.1) made up of a number of characteristics that separate professions from other occupations. Professions, according to Hall, are divided into two parts: structure and attitude.

Structure

This relates to formal education and entry requirements and has been explored extensively by Wilensky (1964). The following steps are needed to establish a profession and relate to the structure (Wilensky, 1964):

- A full-time occupation is one which necessitates specific knowledge, skills and functions, many of which relate to the needs of the society it is serving;
- A training school is established and a knowledge base organized. This then leads to an affiliation with a university;
- From these criteria professional organizations are formed. At this stage the occupational title may also be changed as attempts are made to define clearly the exact nature of the profession and to specify the tasks executed;
- A code of ethics is then devised relating to internal (colleagues) and external (society) individuals. The code is enforced by the profession.

Attitudinal components

According to Hall (1968) these comprise:

- Ideas and judgements which are produced as a direct result of formal and informal group decisions within the profession;
- A belief, which is held by the profession, that a service is provided to the public: work performed by the profession benefits the public and practitioner;
- The profession is viewed by its members as being essential to society;
- The belief that members have a vocation and that the professional person is dedicated to her work;
- The view that the profession is autonomous and free to make its decisions and judgements.

Points for discussion:

- Discuss these statements.

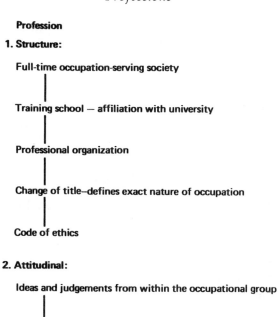

Profession

1. Structure:

Full-time occupation-serving society

Training school — affiliation with university

Professional organization

Change of title–defines exact nature of occupation

Code of ethics

2. Attitudinal:

Ideas and judgements from within the occupational group

Belief by occupation — service to public

Belief by occupation — essential to society

Occupational members — sense of calling

Autonomy

Figure 1.1 Professional model (Hall, 1968).

- Relate these statements to nursing.

Hall (1968) worked with various professional groups, including a group of American nurses from a private general hospital. The results he obtained from his investigation of their views suggested that:

- Nurses had a strong belief that they were providing a service for the public;
- They had a 'sense of calling';
- Autonomy was affected by the nurse's position within the hospital hierarchy. They felt that having to follow and

recognize medical practice and policies created a degree of conflict with nursing practice and the professional code, thus reducing their autonomy.

Points for discussion:

- Could these findings be related to nurses in Britain?
- Could the views be applicable to nurses working in A and E?

Functionalist model

Rueschemeyer (1983) describes the **functionalist model of professionalism** in the following terms:

- Skills and knowledge, held by experts, which are required by individuals in need of assistance. This is acknowledged by the individuals who need immediate help as well as by those who may need such skills and knowledge in the future;

Points for discussion:

- Discuss the words 'skills', 'knowledge', 'experts' as used in this statement.
- Individuals outside the profession accept that specialist skills and knowledge lead to the provision of a service. Inability to gain access to such skills and knowledge ensures that these cannot be evaluated;

Points for discussion:

- Consider A and E nursing, does the above statement apply?
- Experts control experts;

Points for discussion:

- With reference to the above statement, discuss the advantages and disadvantages for those receiving the service.
- A deal is struck with society, competence is given by the profession in exchange for trust in and acceptance of the profession by society;
- The profession enjoys freedom from lay (outside the profession) supervision and interference;

Points for discussion:

- Do these statements apply to A and E nursing? Give reasons to support your answer.
- The profession is allowed to control: recruitment; training; organization; code of ethics; standards and codes enforced through professional courts.

Points for discussion:

- Can nursing be described as a profession?
- Compare your answer with those of your colleagues.

ORGANIZATIONAL THEORY

Weeks (1973) states that 'the organization is a very important mediating institution between the wider societal culture and the individual social actor'. This statement indicates that Weeks thought of an organization as an intermediate establishment linking the individual and society. However, there are numerous types of organizations which can take many forms. For example, the National Health Service (NHS), supermarkets, schools and a charity are all types of organizations. Each has a specific structure, goals, problems, personnel and particular reasons for their existence.

Points for discussion:

- Consider an organization outside the NHS and make a list of its components.
- Discuss how all the identified components contribute to the overall structure of the organization.
- Discuss the organization of the hospital in which you work.
- Compare the organization of the A and E department with that of a ward.

An organization can be defined and described in a variety of ways, and some of the approaches will be discussed below.

Systems approach

This approach views the organization as a whole. Parsons (1956) defined an organization as 'a social system which is organized for the attainment of a particular goal; the attainment of that goal is at the same time the performance of a type of function on behalf of a more inclusive system, the society'.

Points for discussion:

- How can this statement be related to the organization of the A and E department?

It is argued that a system (organization) is present within society to meet particular needs: for example, health and survival needs of the individual or groups of individuals (Salaman and Thompson, 1973). The organization exists to meet specific needs and the requirement of needs to be met ensures the continued existence of the organization. This helps create a mechanism that encourages reduction of conflict within the organization (Weeks, 1973).

Points for discussion:

- Discuss ways in which the needs of society can be measured.
- For what reasons were A and E departments founded?

Universalist approach

This approach examines general principles and techniques of an organization; arrangement of work, incentives and rewards for the workforce (Weeks, 1973).

Taylor (1970), the pioneer of scientific management, advocated the universalist approach. General principles were explored while the individual feelings of workers were often disregarded (Tosi, 1984).

Particularist approach

The particularist approach argues that different organizations face different problems, such as those associated with people within the organization, machinery or the environment. For this reason it is difficult to produce general theories. Instead, specific aspects of the organization should be examined.

Points for discussion:

- Consider the universalist and particularist approaches to organizations. Do one, both or none apply to the organization of the A and E department.
- Give reasons for your answer.

Tosi (1984) views the examination of an organization as the study of a system, a view held by Parsons (1956). Tosi breaks down the system into different parts and examines these. Reference is made to other research in this area (March and Simon, 1958; Henderson, 1953; Haire, 1959) and this is cited in support of his study of organizations.

According to Barnard (1938), an organization is formed when individuals begin to communicate with each other and are willing to act to achieve a commonly defined goal.

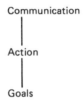

Davis (1951) describes an organization as a collection of individuals led by one person. Their aim is to meet a particular goal. However, Stogdill (1959) describes organizations in terms of behaviour and roles. His model has its roots in social psychology. A similar view is expressed by Cummings (1978) who sees an organization as the result of individual and group behaviour.

Points for discussion:

- How would you define an organization?

Organizational components

According to Scott (1961), an organization can be disseminated into different parts and these components are discussed below.

The individual

Comprising of a complex personality, motives, values and attitudes, the individual will participate within the system for a selection of reasons and will also have her own personal goals.

The formal organization

Within the formal organization there will be a specific range of activities, including tasks and supervision. The individual may have expectations and goals related to the jobs she is expected to do, and there may be conflict between personal goals and those of the organization (Argyris, 1957).

The informal organization

This refers to the interaction of particular groups of individuals within the organization. Such interaction is responsible for the modification of the individual's behaviour. The individual also has expectations about belonging to a group, receiving and giving support, and about friendship.

Role demands and role perception

Both of these have their roots in the formal and informal strands of the organization. To survive and function adequately within an organization, an individual may need to modify her role. Bakke (1959) explores role expectations within organizations, and found that adjustment of individual roles may be necessary in order to enable the organization to survive.

The physical setting

The environment in which specific jobs are performed by individuals is another component of the organization. There is the general environment and there may be special areas set aside for jobs that require technical skills or those in which people work with machinery. Such job content and interaction may affect an individual's role, relationships and other types of interaction within the organization.

Points for discussion:

- Take each component, as described by Scott (1961), and discuss it in relation to the A and E department.
- Can the A and E department be divided into similar components?

The linking process

Three important activities – communication, balance and decision-making – are necessary if all components of the organization, as described above, are to be linked (Tosi, 1984).

Communication can be described as both formal or informal (Chapter 4), and there is communication between peer groups or through the hierarchy. It is important to explore such communication networks as these are crucial elements to any organization.

Points for discussion:

- Consider the research that has been done on communication in the NHS in general and in nursing in particular and describe the methods used.
- Which types of communication are used in A and E?
- How do you evaluate the effectiveness of communication within the A and E department?
- Apart from the passage of information, what other uses does communication have?

Individual sectors of organizations must communicate with each other as well as with agencies outside the organization. Each part receives information from the outside world and stores this information (Deutsch, 1952).

The second linking activity is balance. The various components of the organization create relationships with each other, the goal being the stability of the whole organization. Upset of the balance could result in destruction of the organization. Balance is also necessary to facilitate change within an organization.

Changes within an organization can create difficulties and most will have specific methods to deal with change. These may include various communication techniques, modified techniques and jobs, movement of individuals.

In some cases, it may be necessary to employ specialized techniques to cope with change. Also, new or adopted forms of communication may be required to deal with information about new working techniques and jobs. Change will relocate particular components within the organization which could affect the balance. Therefore, the aim is to achieve new relationships so that the stability of the organization can be re-established.

Points for discussion:

- Consider some changes that have affected the whole A and E department.
- How were the various components affected?
- How was the balance re-established?

In order to maintain the balance of an organization during the change process, the following points should be considered (Tosi, 1984).

- Can the organization supply information to individuals about the proposed change within the organization?
- Are components within the organization able to utilize information?
- Are there rules that control the accurate relaying of information to the correct areas within the organization?
- Is provision made for the organization to adjust to change?

It may be necessary for new strategies to be developed to deal with new methods, as the old ones may not be appropriate (Figure 1.2).

Points for discussion:

- Consider how you deal with change.
- What effect does this have on your clinical practice?
- How is change dealt with by others in the A and E department?

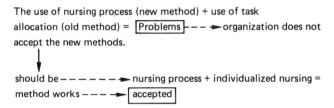

The use of nursing process (new method) + use of task allocation (old method) = Problems - - - ➤ organization does not accept the new methods.

should be - - - - - - ➤ nursing process + individualized nursing = method works - - - ➤ accepted

Figure 1.2 An example of new strategies for the provision of change.

- Consider the methods available within the A and E department to deal with change.

The third linking process is decision-making, which was viewed by Tosi (1984) as the result of individual attitudes and the demands of the organization.

An individual's decision to participate within an organization may be based on a number of different factors. These include motivation, rewards and an awareness of what is available outside that particular organization (March and Simon, 1958). Decisions by individuals are also made within the organization. These relate to jobs, machinery, the consumer, the product, change and the introduction of new methods (Marschak, 1959).

The recognition and use of decision-making maintains the relationship between the numerous components within the organization, and, depending on the success of the decision-making, the organization can succeed or fail.

Points for discussion:

- Describe the decision-making process in A and E.

Configuration of an organization

An organization assumes a particular configuration based upon the arrangement of its components (Mintzberg, 1979). The arrangement will be affected by the amount of power held by a component and its relationship to other components within the organization. Configuration of an organization is also dependent upon its overall structure, age, size and the environment within which it functions (Figure 1.3).

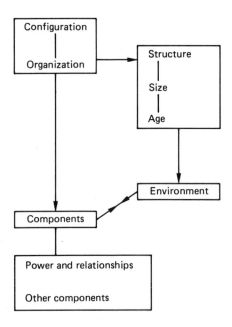

Figure 1.3   Configuration of an organization.

Mintzberg (1979) divided the organization into four co-ordinating parts which are used to segregate and coordinate individuals and labour.

Direct supervision

Mintzberg discusses direct supervision when one individual is responsible for organizing the work of others. Orders are given directly to other individuals. Work is then supervised and coordinated.

Points for discussion:

- Discuss the use of direct supervision in the A and E department.

Standardization of work processes

This is achieved when the job, tasks and other forms of work are specified; rules are established and followed.

Points for discussion:

- Describe the advantages and disadvantages of standardization in A and E nursing.

Standardization of outputs

Standardization of outputs can be achieved when the results of the work are specified, and when particular outcomes are demanded. However, the individual may have freedom to use a variety of methods to achieve the specified outcomes.

Points for discussion:

- Which parts of your clinical practice depend upon standardized outcomes?

Standardization of skills

This is achieved when specific training is required before specified work can be undertaken.

Points for discussion:

- Discuss ways in which communication may be affected by standardization of nursing skills.

Specific parts of an organization

Mintzberg (1979) described the specific parts of an organization (Figure 1.4).

The operating core

This is the lowest tier of the organization, and individuals within this layer perform basic tasks. Usually these tasks are directly related to the production of a service or a product.

The strategic apex

The strategic apex is at the top of the organization, and individuals located here ensure that the organization supplies a service in the most effective way. They must also

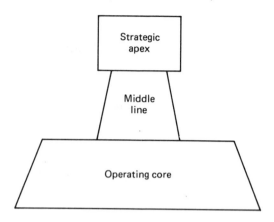

Figure 1.4   Specific parts of an organization.

negotiate with people who control or have power over the organization (government agencies, unions of employees, pressure groups).

The middle line

This layer joins the strategic apex to the operating core. Employees in this layer are referred to as managers or supervisors. The functions of this group include the feedback and upward communication of information, control of the environment and allocation of predefined resources. The individual's specific place within this layer determines the type of tasks performed. Those nearer the operating core have more structured work, those nearer the strategic apex less structured.

Points for discussion:

* Describe the layers of the organization within the A and E department.

The professional bureaucracy (Figure 1.5)

Mintzberg (1979) makes a few points in relation to professional bureaucracy:

* The operating core is made up of professionals and is the most significant layer of the organization;

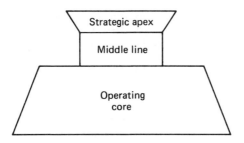

Figure 1.5 The professional bureaucracy.

- The professional has much more control over her work than other individuals and often works closely with the recipient of the service;
- Coordination is accomplished through standardization of skills;
- Standardization occurs following training and indoctrination. Professionals are trained by institutions other than by the employing authority. Therefore, standards are set by the professions outside the organization.

In this chapter, there have been arguments, problems and questions raised which the reader has been encouraged to examine critically, with special reference to their own work setting and to A and E nursing. Further issues will be raised in the following chapters with a view to continued discussion and analysis.

REFERENCES

Argyris, C. (1957) *Personality and organisation* (New York: Harper Brothers).

Bakke, E.W. (1959) 'Concept of the social organisation', in M. Haire, *Modern organisational theory* (New York: John Wiley and Sons).

Barnard, C. (1938) 'The functions of the executive' in G. Salaman and K. Thompson (1973), *People and organisations* (London: Longman for Open University Press).

Carr-Saunders, A.M. (1928) *Professions: Their organisations and place in society* (Oxford: Clarendon Press).

Caplow, T.A. (1954) *The sociology of work* (Minneapolis: University of Minnesota Press).

Cummings, L.L. (1978) 'Towards organisational behaviour', *J. Acad. Manag. Rev.*, vol. 3, no. 1, pp. 90–8.

Davis, R.C. (1951) *The fundamentals of top management* (New York: Harper Brothers).

Deutsch, K.W. (1952) 'On communication models in social sciences', *Pub. Opin. Quart.*, vol. 16, pp. 356–80.

Dingwell, R. (1976) 'Accomplishing profession', *Soc. Rev.* vol. 24, pp. 331–49.

Dingwell, R. and Lewis, P. (1983) *The sociology of professions* (London: Macmillan Press Ltd).

Elliot, P. (1972) *The sociology of professions* (London: Macmillan Press Ltd).

Fitzpatrick, J. and Whall, A. (1983) *Conceptual models of nursing, analysis and application* (London: Prentice Hall International Inc).

Friedson, E. (1970) *Profession of medicine: A study of sociology of applied knowledge* (New York: Dodd, Mead & Company).

Friedson, E. (1983) 'The theory of professions: State of the Art', in R. Dingwell and P. Lewis (1983), *The sociology of professions* (London: Macmillan Press Ltd).

Hall, R.H. (1968) 'Professionalisation and Bureaucratisation', *Am. Sociol. Rev.*, vol. 33, pp. 231–6.

Henderson, L.J. (1953) *Pareto's general sociology* (Cambridge: Harvard University Press).

Haire, M. (ed.) (1959) *Modern organisational theory* (New York: John Wiley and Son).

Illich, I. (1977) *Disabling professions* (London: Marion Boyars).

Johnson, T.J. (1972) *Professions and power* (London: Macmillan Press Ltd).

Larson, M.S. (1977) *The rise of professionalism: A sociological analysis* (London: University of California Press).

Laski, H.L. (1931) 'The limitations of the expert', in R. Dingwell and P. Lewis (1983), *The sociology of professions* (London: Macmillan Press Ltd).

March, G. and Simon, H. (1958) *Organisations* (New York: John Wiley).

Marschak, J. (1959) 'Efficient and viable organisational forms', in M. Haire (1959), *Modern organisational theory* (New York: John Wiley and Sons).

McCormack, J. (1979) *The doctor: father figure or plumber* (London: Croom Helm).

Mintzberg, H. (1979) *The structuring of organisations* (New Jersey, Englewood Cliffs: Prentice Hall).

Parsons, T. (1956) 'Suggestions for a sociological approach to the theory of organisations', in G. Salaman and K. Thompson (1973), *People and organisations* (London: Longman for Open University Press).

Roper, N., Logan, W.W. and Tierney, A. (1983) *Using a model for nursing* (Edingburgh: Churchill Livingstone).

Rueschemeyer D. (1983) 'Professional autonomy and the social control of expertise', in R. Dingwell and P. Lewis (1983), *The sociology of professions* (London: Macmillan Press Ltd).

Salaman, G. and Thompson, K. (1973) *People and organisations* (London: Longman for the Open University Press).

Salvage, J. and Kershaw, B. (1990) *Models for nursing* 2 (London: Scutari Press).

Scott, W. (1961) 'Organisational theory', *J. Acad. Manag.*, vol. 4, no. 1, pp. 7–26.

Stogdill, R.M. (1959) *Individual behaviour and group achievement* (Oxford: Oxford University Press).

Taylor, F.W. (1970) 'Scientific management,' in G. Salaman and K. Thompson (1973), *People and organisations* (London: Longman for Open University Press).

Tosi, H.L. (1984) *Theories of organisations* (2nd ed.) (New York: John Wiley and Sons).

Vollmer, H.W. and Mills, D.J. (eds) (1966) *Professionalization* (New Jersey: Prentice Hall).

Weeks, D. (1973) '*Organisation theory-some themes and distinctions'*, in G. Salaman and K. Thompson (1973), *People and organisations* (London: Longman for Open University Press).

Wilensky, H.L. (1964) 'The professionalisation of everyone', *Am. J. Soc.*, vol. 70, pp. 142–6.

Wright, S.G. (1986) *Building and using a model of nursing* (London: Edward Arnold).

Chapter 2

A philosophical framework for nursing care in the A and E department

CONTENTS

INTRODUCTION

To understand a whole subject it is often easier to break it down into its different components and then to examine these in detail. In chapters 2 and 3 the aim is to do this with the discipline of philosophy. Through the use of discussion points the reader is invited to examine the relevant issues and then to apply these to her clinical practice. After a general introduction to the subject, there will be a brief review of values, attitudes and language.

The development of a philosophical framework for nursing care in the A and E department will be continued in Chapter 3 as the implications for practice are examined further in that section.

WHAT IS PHILOSOPHY?

'Most human beings are curious . . . they want to find out about the world around them and about their part in this world' (Emmet, 1968). The discipline of philosophy has evolved from this type of curiosity.

O'Hear (1985) views philosophy as a rational and systematic questioning of everything with which human beings come into contact. Individuals want to ask questions, to wonder and to speculate (Emmet, 1968). Philosophy encompasses attempts by individuals and society to answer questions about the environment and other aspects of life.

The word 'philosophy' is derived from the Greeks and relates to the love of knowledge and wisdom. Aristotle, who is regarded as one of the greatest philosophers, demonstrated this by asking questions and speculating about many issues including politics and science, illustrating that, at this time, philosophy included most fields of knowledge. As technology and research into various areas have advanced, many of the original questions, such as those relating to chemistry, have been satisfactorily answered. Thus, the resulting body of knowledge has been incorporated into another discipline. For example, chemistry has left the discipline of philosophy and is now associated with the discipline of science.

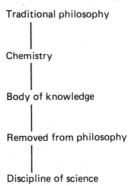

Traditional philosophy

Chemistry

Body of knowledge

Removed from philosophy

Discipline of science

There still are, however, many subjects which require considerable thought and that still have no satisfactory answers, and philosophers continue to explore these. Although, nowadays, philosophy is divided up into different areas of investigation. For example, the study of problems primarily concerned with how individuals use thinking and argument is called logic. Another branch of philosophy is epistemology; the study of knowledge. This involves the study of what individuals claim to know or believe they know. The study of morals and rules of behaviour is called ethics.

In all areas, the philosopher is interested in investigating the roots of the subject or problem rather than the outcome. The goal is a complete picture of what an individual thinks and knows (Popkin and Stroll, 1989).

Warnock (1958), a modern philosopher, views the discipline as being concerned with ideas, the ways in which they are organized by the individual and communicated to others. The question asked has taken on more importance in modern philosophy than its answer. The attempt to view problems objectively is the basis of philosophizing (Emmet, 1968; Popkin and Stroll, 1989).

The term philosophy has also come to mean other things in today's society: an attitude towards certain activities, analysis of what is important, placing things in perspective (Popkin and Stroll, 1989).

Points for discussion:

- Describe how you have used the term philosophy in the past.
- How do others use the term philosophy?

VALUES

The study of values is generally associated with the study of man (Reich and Adcock, 1976), although work done in this area reflects varied views. Values may be considered of little (Skinner, 1971) or of considerable (Rokeach, 1973) significance.

Jones and Gerard (1967) state that 'any singular state or object for which the individual strives or approaches, extols, embraces, voluntarily consumes, incurs expense to acquire is a positive value ... Values animate the person, they move him around his environment because they define its attractive and repelling sections'.

Individuals aim for that which they consider to be of value to them.

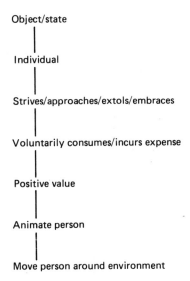

Object/state

|

Individual

|

Strives/approaches/extols/embraces

|

Voluntarily consumes/incurs expense

|

Positive value

|

Animate person

|

Move person around environment

Points for discussion:

- Discuss this statement in relation to you.
- Describe what you believe constitutes a value.
- Are values interchangeable:
  between individuals?
  between the individual and society?
  between societies?

As values cannot be observed directly (Reich and Adcock, 1976), there may be problems when individuals attempt to describe them.

Points for discussion:

- Consider one value that you hold and describe this to another person.
- How simple/complicated was this to do?

A value held by one individual may correspond or conflict with a value held by another. Therefore, problems may be encountered by both individuals as they attempt to describe their own values and those of the other person.

Points for discussion:

- Within a small group, choose a value familiar to all parties and discuss this.

There are degrees of values, or layers (Reich and Adcock, 1976), and Tschudin (1986) describes a hierarchy of values. For example, values relating to life and death may be placed within a hierarchy or 'weighed' against other values.

Points for discussion:

• Consider your hierarchy of values.

Values are not independent of the person and this may lead to the inability of the person to view objectively or to discuss particular values relating to her.

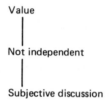

In addition to their previous definition (p. 24), Jones and Gerard (1967) continue their description of what is meant by a value. They feel that it results from 'a relationship between a person's emotional feelings and particular cognitive categories'.

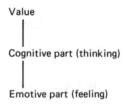

Values are made up of two components: one thinking, one feeling. Both components are required before a value is said to be present within an individual. It is not enough to think or have knowledge about a particular object or person, there has to be a feeling attached to the thought. The accompanying feeling can usually be described as positive or negative. In relation to this, Rokeach (1973) gives values an enduring quality as well. He views values as sustained beliefs in the desirability of a particular action or outcome: such a decision follows rejections of other known actions or outcomes. This definition allows for the emotional component of a value; the experience of good or bad feelings connected with the identified object or state. With reference to the word belief, Tschudin (1986) states that this is a basic value that is less susceptible to change.

Points for discussion:

- Discuss the following phrases: negative value;
                                              no value;
                                              valueless;
                                              positive value.
- Discuss the statement: 'nursing is a valuable job'.
- How do you decide that something is of value to you?
- Has society a role in determining your value system?
- Do such questions and arguments have anything to do with the practice of nursing in A and E?

It is essential that individuals scrutinize their personal values so that they can become self aware. This, in turn, could lead to significance being placed upon those values specifically associated with clinical practice. Tschudin (1986) states that self awareness is a useful beginning in the understanding of others. Thought and discussion about values and beliefs can be considered the first step towards the formulation of a nursing philosophy.

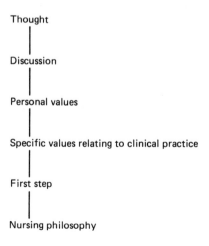

Thought

Discussion

Personal values

Specific values relating to clinical practice

First step

Nursing philosophy

Points for discussion:

- Which positive aspects of clinical practice do you consider relate to your values?
- Consider the above question, replacing positive with negative.
- Describe how you may benefit from an awareness of your values.

Many values only become significant when tested against someone or something (Tschudin, 1986).

Points for discussion: Try the following exercise within a group of a least three people

- Name three things relating to your job that you consider are of value: to you; to your colleagues within the group.
- Name three things that patients attending an A and E department would consider of value.
  Put the answers into a container. Then, each person in the group should pull out one answer, read it and then try to guess to which category, colleague or patient, the answer belongs.
- Discuss your findings within the group.

A discussion about values might include an examination of the outcomes of specific values. The following is an example of how a discussion about the value *equality* leads to statements about patient care.

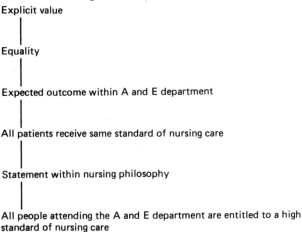

Explicit value

Equality

Expected outcome within A and E department

All patients receive same standard of nursing care

Statement within nursing philosophy

All people attending the A and E department are entitled to a high standard of nursing care

Points for discussion:

• Discuss the implications for clinical practice of making such values explicit within a nursing philosophy.

Discussion among nurses in the A and E department will invariably lead to decisions and statements that affect clinical practice. Although individual nurses may be able to readily identify with the value of **equality**, the purpose of a nursing philosophy is to identify and make known to all, such values within a group. The implications of this may be that group pressure could and often does influence patient care.

Points for discussion:

• Compare the actions of (i) a group and (ii) an individual in relation, to the possible outcomes for patient care.
• How can group values be realized?

Finally, values are considered motivational to the individual. Allport (1961) views values as beliefs which a person acts upon through choice. This is supported by other work (Reich and Adcock, 1976; Rokeach, 1973), which advocates the view that values are motivational.

To use, once again, the value of **equality**, it could be argued that this value would motivate a nurse to provide a high standard of nursing care for *all* patients, rather than differential care for specific groups. Associated with their motivational properties, values act as standards; principles that individuals aim to achieve (Rokeach, 1973).

Points for discussion:

• Discuss the use of values as standards.
• Relate this to clinical practice in A and E.

By achieving the outcome of a high standard of care for all people attending A and E, certain needs within the nurse and patient should be met (Rokeach, 1973). The nurse, through achieving her goal, may meet her self esteem needs (Maslow, 1971). In addition, it could be argued that the patient would also have a variety of needs met: physical, psychological, social, cultural and religious. Recognition of such needs, however, is another subject for debate and is addressed later in this book.

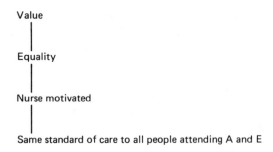

Value

Equality

Nurse motivated

Same standard of care to all people attending A and E

As previously discussed, values have a lasting quality (Rokeach, 1973). It should be emphasized, therefore, that any attempt to modify the values and beliefs of others may present formidable problems. As has already been shown, values are held at both cognitive and emotive levels. Therefore, an individual who has invested in a particular value may be reluctant to surrender it easily. It will be necessary for that person to reinvest emotional and cognitive energy in order to reassign and recategorize specific values.

Points for discussion:

- Describe how values in others may be altered.
- Describe problems that may be encountered.

ATTITUDES

There is a close relationship between values and attitudes. Invariably, therefore, discussion of one will lead to discussion of the other. An awareness of personal attitudes through thought and discussion should generate self awareness and an appreciation of attitudes held by other people.

Points for discussion:

- Consider your definition of an attitude.
- Describe the relationship between your definition and A and E nursing.

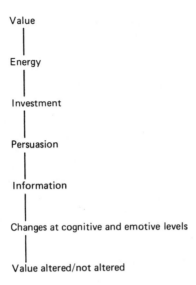

Value

Energy

Investment

Persuasion

Information

Changes at cognitive and emotive levels

Value altered/not altered

In his definition of attitudes, Kelvin (1969) stated that 'man can only cope with his environment if that environment is reasonably orderly and predictable, so that the individual and group in society may know where they stand and what

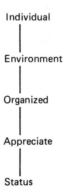

Individual

Environment

Organized

Appreciate

Status

to do'. In other words, attitudes are a necessary prerequisite for an individual to appreciate her relationship to that environment.

Kelvin argued that the environment could be organized by identifying particular values and attitudes and by acting upon these. He felt that organized thoughts, feelings and subsequent actions fostered survival of the individual within a particular setting. This, he argued, ensures that the individual does not have to assess constantly her environment before choosing to act. Through the use of attitudes, certain stimuli produce certain responses.

Attitudes are made up of three main components: affective, cognitive and conative (Reich and Adcock, 1976). This can be illustrated, for example, in relation to professional self development. If the individual feels positive towards self development, this is the *affective* component, and positive knowledge about self development is the *cognitive* part. However, any action related to the above is not part of the attitude. It is the *tendency to act* that should be considered when referring to attitudes. Attitudes, like values, cannot be directly observed (Atkinson *et al*, 1987). The action associated with the feeling and thoughts cannot be part of an attitude for actions that can be directly observed.

Points for discussion:

- Discuss the difference between action and the tendency to act in relation to attitudes.
- Take one of your attitudes and break it down into the three components (affective, cognitive and tendency to act).

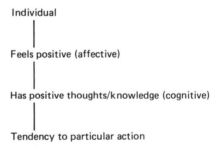

Individual

Feels positive (affective)

Has positive thoughts/knowledge (cognitive)

Tendency to particular action

Krech, Cruchfield and Ballachey (1962) view attitudes as 'enduring systems of positive or negative evaluations, emotional feelings, and pro or con action techniques with respect to social objects. Attitudes are specific appraisals of the environment and are associated with particular actions'.

Points for discussion:

- Discuss the use of the word 'enduring' in relation to attitudes.
- Relate this to clinical practice in A and E.

'An attitude is a predisposition to experience, to be motivated by, and to act toward, a class of objects in a predictable manner' (Smith, Bruner and White, 1956).

Points for discussion:

- Discuss the use of the term 'motivated' in connection with attitudes.
- Relate this to clinical practice in A and E.
- Discuss the following:
  Consistency between beliefs and attitudes is a common occurrence in life;
  To believe in something or someone usually has a positive attitude attached to it (Atkinson *et al*, 1987).
- Consider the part played by attitudes when formulating a nursing philosophy.

USE OF LANGUAGE AND COMMUNICATION IN PHILOSOPHY

The use of language as a medium should be the subject of all philosophical studies (Emmet, 1968). As thoughts and ideas can only be analyzed and discussed through the use of language, care is necessary in the choice of words for these need to be understood by all involved parties. However, the use of language is taken for granted by many people (Emmet, 1968) and, although the majority of individuals use it, most do not consider its use. It is often only when a person attempts to learn a new language that the implications of the use of language are understood. On such occasions the use of language may suddenly become very frustrating as communication problems can result from the wrong usage of words.

Points for discussion:

- Discuss the use of language as a medium for thinking and speaking.

- Consider your use of written and spoken language in relation to your work.

Language has two aspects: production and comprehension (Atkinson *et al*, 1987). In the use of language we have a thought, we then produce a sound which is developed into a word and then a sentence. This process involves both the production and comprehension of language.

Points for discussion:

- What is thinking?

According to the Collins English Dictionary, to think is to have one's mind at work, reflect, meditate, reason, deliberate, imagine, hold opinion. However, Emmet (1968) makes the distinction between thinking and verbal communication as that of private communication (thinking) and public communication (speaking). Language is required to ensure that access to others' thoughts can be obtained.

Points for discussion:

- What relevance does the awareness of thoughts and language have to your communication skills?
- What does communication involve?

The communication process involves style, appearance and body movement (Janner, 1988). This includes the projection of voice, warmth, sincerity, eye contact and the use of active listening.

Points for discussion:

- During your last conversation, estimate the time spent speaking and that spent listening.
- Think about a person that you consider to be a good communicator. Why do you view them in this way?

Language is necessary for individuals to make thoughts, ideas, beliefs, values and attitudes explicit within a group, such as nurses in A and E. This should, therefore, be considered an important aspect of formulating a nursing philosophy. It will also form an important part of communicating that philosophy to others at a later date, as people exposed to a written nursing philosophy should be able to understand it. Patients and their families may be some of the people wishing to be informed about the departmental philosophy. For this reason, the use of clear, concise statements is important. To achieve this goal, the use of words should be carefully considered, and the use of jargon, specialized language, and the use of pretentious or nonsensical language should be eliminated. This is important as the interpretation of such words could lead to misunderstanding.

Points for discussion:

- Consider the following words: wild, disturbance, careful, good, nice.
- How many meanings can you attach to these particular words?
  NB. Reference to a dictionary and thesaurus will illustrate the number of meanings available.

As already stated, language is an important medium for transmitting thoughts (Emmet, 1968). Such thoughts relating to A and E nursing may need careful translation into concise statements.

This chapter has introduced the reader to various components that may be found within philosophical frameworks for nursing care. Chapter 3 continues with the theme and examines the implications for practice within the A and E department.

REFERENCES

Allport, G.W. (1961) *Pattern and growth in personality* (New York: Holt, Rinehart & Winston).

Atkinson, R.L., Atkinson, R., Smith, E.E. and Hilgard, E.R. (1987) *Introduction to psychology* (9th ed.) (London: Harcourt Brace Jovanovich Publishers).

Collins English Dictionary (1989) (London: Collins)

Emmet, E.R. (1968) *Learning to philosophize* (Harmondsworth: Penguin).

Janner, G. (1988) *Janner on communication* (London: Hutchinson Business Books).

Jones, E.E. and Gerard, H.B. (1967) *Foundation of social psychology* (New York: John Wiley).

Kelvin, P. (1969) *The basis of social behaviour* (New York: Holt, Rinehart & Winston).

Krech, D., Crutchfield, R.A. and Ballachy, E.L. (1962) *Individual in society: a textbook of social psychology* (New York: McGraw Hill).

Maslow, A.H. (1971) *Motivation and personality* (2nd ed.) (London: Harper and Row).

O'Hear, A. (1985) *What philosophy is – an introduction to contemporary philosophy* (Harmondsworth: Penguin).

Popkin, R.H. and Stroll, A. (1989) *Philosophy* (2nd ed.) (London: Heinemann).

Reich, B. and Adcock, C. (1976) *Values, attitudes & behaviour change* (London: Methuen).

Rokeach, M. (1973) *The nature of human values* (New York: Free Press).

Skinner, B.F. (1971) *Beyond freedom and dignity* (New York: Knopf).

Smith, H.B., Bruner, J.S. and White, R.W. (1956) *Opinions and personality* (New York: John Wiley).

Tschudin, V. (1986) *Ethics in nursing, the caring relationship* (London: Heinemann).

Warnock, G.J. (1958) 'English philosophy since 1900', in E.R. Emmet (1968), *Learning to philosophize* (Harmondsworth: Penguin).

FURTHER READING

Hossack, A. (1973) *Express yourself with power* (Guildford: Lutterworth Press).

Nagel, T. (1987) *What does it all mean? (Philosophy)* (Oxford: Oxford University Press).

Chapter 3

A philosophical framework for nursing care: implications for practice

CONTENTS

- Introduction
- Concepts
- Knowledge: definition and use
- Constructing a nursing philosophy
- Uses of a nursing philosophy
- Nursing philosophies and nursing models
- References
- Further reading

INTRODUCTION

Values, beliefs, attitudes and the use of language were discussed in Chapter 2, and further components of philosophy; concepts and knowledge will be examined in this chapter. After this, a philosophical framework for nursing care will be discussed with special emphasis on its relevance to clinical practice within the A and E department. Once again, the reader is invited to investigate the application of such ideas to her own nursing practice through the use of discussion points.

CONCEPTS

The term concept may be used in connection with the formulation of nursing philosophies. It is variously described as an idea, impression, theory (Collins Thesaurus, 1989), and as a mental expression or abstract idea (Collins English Dictionary, 1989). A concept can be associated with most ideas that an individual may have, and these ideas may or may not have been discussed in conversation and measured against other people's concepts. Concepts provide a way of dividing the world into manageable units (Atkinson *et al*, 1987).

Points for discussion:

- Discuss the concept of a nursing philosophy.
- Are individuals aware of concepts within their minds?

Concepts relate to how an individual sees an aspect of her life, the impression in her mind. For example, the concept of going on holiday. This involves the mental impression a person has of her next holiday. At this stage, it is a concept – the impressions are in her mind, the event has not yet happened. However, once the holiday is undertaken it becomes part of reality. It may or may not compare with the individual's original concept of how the holiday would be.

In some cases, there may be knowledge associated with the subject. For example, the production of electricity creates ideas and impressions in a person's head: concepts. In nursing practice, there are concepts that require exploration, such as home visits from A and E nurses. In relation to these concepts, there may be little or conflicting information available. For example, there are concepts about rare diseases about which there may only be limited information, and there are ideas about life after death which can be conflicting.

Points for discussion:

- Think about a type of food you have never tasted, what is your concept of this food?
- From where have you obtained these concepts?

It can be seen from this and the previous discussion (Chapter 2) that beliefs, values and attitudes could be expressed within the framework of a concept. Language is the medium through which thoughts and ideas can be shared and made explicit. However, before this is related to nursing philosophies there is a further issue that must be covered: knowledge.

KNOWLEDGE: DEFINITION AND USE

To state that something is known by an individual implies that what is known is believed and what is believed is true. Such knowledge cannot include that which a person believes but without good reason and that which the person believes but which turns out to be false (O'Hear, 1985).

Points for discussion:

- How do you determine what is true and what is false?
- What relevance has such a statement to A and E nursing?

If nurses are to examine their beliefs, values and attitudes in relation to A and E nursing and become aware of what ideas they hold, they may reach a point when they begin to question what it is they know. To examine what is known about nursing, the people using A and E services and colleagues, nurses in A and E must question how such knowledge has been acquired.

Points for discussion:

- How did you acquire your knowledge about A and E nursing?
- Of what is this knowledge comprised?
- Consider regular attenders at the A and E department.
  Do you know why they attend?
  Do you believe they attend for particular reasons?
  Compare your answer with those of your colleagues.

O'Hear (1985) suggests that there are two broad types of knowledge: knowledge by acquaintance and knowledge by description. **Knowledge by acquaintance** is that knowledge acquired through personal experience. **Knowledge by description** is the acquisition of facts through verbal accounts.

Points for discussion:

- Through which method, by acquaintance or by description, did you acquire (a) your knowledge about nursing and (b) your knowledge about nursing models?

Philosophers remain concerned about what individuals know or think they know (Popkin and Stroll, 1989). This introduces the term opinion, which is defined by the Collins English Dictionary (1989) as 'what one thinks about something, belief, judgement'. Some philosophers have stated that people's knowledge only expresses opinion which may or may not be true (Popkin and Stroll, 1989). Others claim that there is obtainable information that is not mere opinion but which is unquestionably true.

Points for discussion:

- With reference to this definition, can an opinion still be considered knowledge?

Points for discussion: the photograph and picture exercise
A group of at least three people are needed for this exercise

- Choose a colour photograph of scenery;
- look at a photograph for 30 seconds;
- put the photograph face down;
- each person describes (a) the main feature in the photograph and (b) the second most important feature.
- Do all the descriptions match?
- In what ways do they match?
- In what ways do the descriptions vary?

The discipline of philosophy has been asking questions about knowledge and its acquisition for many years. The purpose of introducing the subject here is to consider knowledge that A and E nurses have, and how this may be incorporated into a nursing philosophy. As stated already, attempts to examine what it is that A and E nurses know and believe may raise questions about what is known and from where this knowledge is obtained.

CONSTRUCTING A NURSING PHILOSOPHY

Values, beliefs, attitudes and language were discussed in Chapter 2, and concepts and knowledge have been examined in this chapter. With this in mind, the reader is invited to discuss the following points in preparation for the formulation of a nursing philosophy.

Points for discussion:

- How do nurses' values relate to clinical practice?

- What do you consider to be the reasons for patients attending A and E departments?
- How does this relate to nurses' attitudes?
- How do nurses' attitudes relate to clinical practice?
- Consider actions that may form part of an attitude.
- Describe the attitudes displayed by patients towards nursing care.
- Consider your attitudes towards other types of nursing e.g. mental health nursing.
- Discuss your concept of nursing as a profession.
- Compare the differences and similarities of your concept with those concepts of your colleagues.
  Consider the public image of A and E, and the origination of this image.
- Compare this to the image given to A and E nursing within the nursing profession.
- With reference to clinical practice, consider the language used by nurses.
- Does speech and expression alter when communicating with patients?.
- Consider the use of jargon and its effects on communication.
- Consider the effects on communication of other types of jargon used in nursing e.g. computer jargon.
- Describe the language used by nurses to describe A and E nursing.

After thought and discussion among nurses within the A and E department, the following questions should be answered:

- What is known about A and E nursing in your department?
- What is known about nursing in other A and E departments?
- What is known about the people who attend A and E departments?
- How has this knowledge been acquired?

Such exploration of A and E nursing should assist in the preparation for the formulation of a nursing philosophy. During discussion, consideration could be given to making a list of key words that describe A and E nursing. This should help readers to organize their thoughts and to highlight similar and conflicting ideas.

Summary of steps leading to the formulation of a nursing philosophy

1. Explore values and beliefs relating to A and E nursing.
2. Explore attitudes.
3. Examine concepts of A and E nursing; nurses and public.
4. Verbal statements are made relating to what is believed and known about A and E nursing.
5. Written statements are made about A and E nursing.

Example of a nursing philosophy

A and E nursing is primarily concerned with nursing assessment and action associated with physiological imbalances. Once the patient is out of danger from these imbalances, the nurse, patient and family can address any other issues they consider important at that time. These may be physical, social, religious or psychological. By doing this, all persons involved in care-giving and receiving are given the opportunity to choose and make decisions relating to care and all that is important is considered.

This example demonstrates how statements about A and E nursing can be made. Statements made within a nursing philosophy should reflect how the nurses view A and E nursing. If this is done, then the philosophy is correct. It should be accessible, easy to read and understand.

USES OF A NURSING PHILOSOPHY

An A and E philosophy should create a mental picture of A and E nursing. In discussion it may be necessary to include who will have access to the philosophy and how often the philosophy should be updated. The nursing philosophy should be reviewed as the environment, nursing staff and specialty change and develop. In this way, it will grow with the people using it.

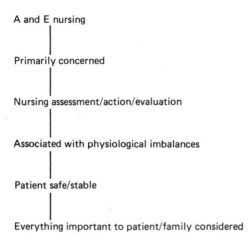

A and E nursing

Primarily concerned

Nursing assessment/action/evaluation

Associated with physiological imbalances

Patient safe/stable

Everything important to patient/family considered

Such statements provide information for both nurses and non-nurses about A and E nurses, and the valuable role of the A and E nurse is defined and communicated to members of the public and the profession as a whole. A nursing philosophy helps to clarify the aims of nurses in the department, and constant reference to it will help individual nurses aim for clearly defined goals. Statements made may refer to what it is the nurses in the department are endeavouring to achieve as well as that which has already been achieved and should now be maintained. As a group of nurses, the philosophy provides a general standard that should be aspired to. It could also, for example, provide a basis for argument about staff shortages and nursing skill mix.

A nursing philosophy may be compared to the colours of an oil painting (Figure 3.1). It is the colours that help create the painting, emphasizing shapes and lines within it. A nursing philosophy helps create a picture of nursing. From the philosophy, ideas are generated. The ideas that such statements generate may be associated with the shapes and lines of the picture. Anyone wishing to understand A and E nursing should be able to obtain a clear picture from a verbal or written nursing philosophy.

This discussion should by now have clarified what comprises a nursing philosophy and how this is translated, through the use of language, into a number of statements.

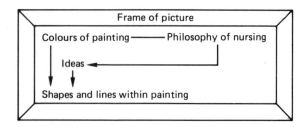

Figure 3.1　Symbolism of a nursing philosophy.

Initially, such statements may be verbal, but eventually written down.

By formulating a nursing philosophy, delving into the minds of the nurses working in A and E and organizing ideas, the concept of A and E nursing will become more explicit.

NURSING PHILOSOPHIES AND NURSING MODELS

Much discussion has now taken place into the formulation and use of nursing philosophies in A and E. Once a philosophy is available the process of selecting a nursing model becomes easier, although it is important to choose one that is sympathetic to the philosophy. In such a nursing model it is necessary to acknowledge and place importance on the quick recognition of physiological imbalances within an individual, as the nature of A and E nursing is often based on quick and accurate decisions. Time cannot be spent trying to fit patient details into an appropriate framework for care. Therefore, the most important requirement is choice of the correct framework.

A nursing model can be defined as a framework for care and this can be compared to the frame of an oil painting (Figure 3.1): it should fit correctly and complement the colours and lines of the painting. A nursing model should be appropriate for the nursing philosophy, otherwise conflict may result.

Points for discussion:

• Consider the implications of choosing a nursing model that is not sympathetic to the nursing philosophy.

- Consider the implications of using a nursing model without first investigating nursing in your department.

One philosophical framework and its implications for practice has now been introduced, and in Chapter 4 there will be exploration of the next phase: the nursing process and nursing models and their application to A and E nursing.

REFERENCES

Atkinson, R.L., Atkinson, R., Smith, E.E. and Hilgard, E.R. (1987) *Introduction to psychology (9th ed.)* (London: Harcourt Brace Jovanovich Publishers).

Collins English Dictionary (1989) (London: Collins).

Collins Thesaurus (1989) (London: Collins).

O'Hear, A. (1985) *What philosophy is – an introduction to contemporary philosophy* (Harmondsworth: Penguin).

Popkin, R.H. and Stroll, A. (1989) *Philosophy* (2nd ed.) (London: Heinemann).

FURTHER READING

Armstrong, S.L., Gleitman, L.R. and Gleitman, H. (1983) 'What some concepts might not be', *Cognition*, vol. 13, pp. 263–308.

Place, B. (1990) 'How to write a ward philosophy', *Nursing Standard*, vol. 4, no. 36, p. 53.

Smith, V.M. and Bass, T.A. (1982) *Communication for the health care team* (Lippincott nursing series) (London: Harper & Row).

Chapter 4

The nursing process in the A and E department

CONTENTS

INTRODUCTION

The use of nursing models, nursing process and documentation in the A and E department will be discussed in this chapter. These will then be related to A and E nursing through the use of examples. The aim of this chapter is to provide information and a basis from which ideas about nursing models in A and E can be developed further by the reader.

The house building process has been included to help define the nursing process. It is hoped that this analogy will aid understanding by providing contrasts and similarities between this and the nursing process.

THE HOUSE BUILDING PROCESS

A house is made up of windows, doors, walls, foundations and a roof. Although this statement is correct, it is doubtful whether a house would remain standing for long, if it were to be built following this sequence of events. In order for a house to be constructed safely, the area where the building is to take place needs to be investigated, and such problems as land movement and other potential building work needs to be identified. Then, the foundations must be dug. These provide the initial strength on which further building takes place. From the foundations walls are built, windows and doors are inserted and a roof added. Omit the foundations and the building is likely to collapse shortly after being constructed. Workmen, therefore, have to follow an organized series of events, to ensure that the building is erected properly and that no stage is omitted.

They must also have the correct building materials and ensure that their tools and equipment are adequate and appropriate for the range of jobs they must perform.

Different workmen should be employed as a skill mix is needed, each worker being able to do a particular number of jobs. For example, some will assess the area, some dig the foundations and others build the walls.

The process of building can, therefore, be described in the following stages.

1. Assessment of:

- Equipment;
- Area;
- Building materials;
- Workers;
- Money.

2. Identification of actual/potential problems:

- Type of land, for example marshy ground;
- Time limit on building;
- Bad weather;
- Financial constrictions.

3. Goals:

- Long-term: to build a house;
- Short-term: to build two walls by summer.

4. Action planning:
This would include a plan of action and desired achievements in a given period of time. For example, taking into consideration the needs of the employer and employees (e.g. holidays), the following goals could be the aim after a four week period from the start of building the house:

- Dig foundations;
- Build one wall;
- Give two men holidays;
- Pay all workmen.

5. Evaluation:

- Building has commenced;
- More workmen are needed;
- There is no money left.

6. Re-assessment necessary.

THE NURSING PROCESS

This can be compared with the house building process for it also needs a foundation from which all planning and action develops. The foundation or *assessment* stage allows for identification of problems relating to the patient (individual), family (social group) and all that surrounds them (environment). This is followed by care planning and nursing action. Should the assessment stage be disregarded the whole process is in danger of collapsing. Problems may be overlooked and subsequent care omitted.

Traditional nursing care relied on identifying and completing a number of tasks. This placed little emphasis on some of the patient's needs and, although patients often consider that nurses are kind, this is not enough. Nurses should be able to understand patients and their families, anticipate their needs and give them continuous support (Wilson–Barnett, 1988).

The nursing process, by advocating early assessment and problem identification, assists in the anticipation of patient needs. Following assessment, goals are set, care is planned, delivered and evaluated. Through these stages patient needs are met.

Patients admitted to A and E departments have various needs: physical, psychological, social, spiritual and cultural. As a client group the emphasis placed on different areas of care may necessitate constant change. Often, there are dramatic changes in their physical condition which may be improving or deteriorating, and psychologically they may be regressing or coping. This results in constantly changing needs of these individuals, which present different problems that require identification and solution. A and E nursing must, therefore, be flexible and take this into account. Use of the nursing process has implications for developing this flexibility, as it would provide a problem solving approach towards the patient and family. This would result in individualized care which could be tailored to suit their needs and altered, if necessary, to accommodate any changes.

The nursing process promotes thought in those who use it. Thinking through the various stages encourages organized planning of individualized care and systematic nursing action. Evaluation aids reflection of action taken. Nurses who can develop this way of thinking are able to use it constantly, during busy periods and when immediate action is needed, thus ensuring that standards of care are maintained. However, the nursing process cannot be used in isolation, it must be linked to a suitable nursing model.

USE OF THE NURSING PROCESS IN A AND E

In considering the use of the nursing process in A and E, it is important to determine which of the following applies to this area of work:

- The nursing process is used;
- The nursing process could be used;
- There is no place for the nursing process;
- No consideration has been given to the use of the nursing process.

Reasons for your answer may be found in the following:

- There is no time available to use such a method;
- It is done but not as described;
- It would not work;
- Do not know;
- Nurses are not needed in A and E so why use the nursing process;
- No-one would read what was written about the patient;
- We will do what we have always done, as this works;
- Patients would not understand;
- Doctors would not like it;
- The role of the A and E nurse should be developing in other ways.

How would your colleagues answer this question? Whatever your answer, the following should be considered.

- How do patients perceive care delivery in A and E?
  Patient care could be improved by enhanced communication.
- Could patient care be improved through the use of the nursing process?
  Patients and their families need to be asked about their perceptions of care.
- How would the nursing process be implemented in A and E?
  The nursing process cannot be implemented in isolation, a nursing model is needed.
- Who could implement it?
  It should be implemented and monitored by those nurses working in the A and E department.
- Does usage of the nursing process have implications for development of the A and E nurse's role?
  Promotion and development of the role of the A and E nurse through the usage of the nursing process should be

investigated, as it is a record of what has been identified, decided and implemented by the A and E nurse.

- Is there any evidence available to support non-usage of the nursing process in the A and E department? Non-usage of the nursing process should be supported by evidence.
- Is the nursing process dismissed because documentation of information is seen as a problem?

THE STAGES OF THE NURSING PROCESS

Assessment

- Information is collected by listening, talking, observing and touching.
- Involvement of patient/family/significant others is necessary if accurate and relevant data are to be acquired in a short space of time.
- Documentation of all information is important and is discussed later in this chapter.

Problem identification

- Actual and potential problems are identified through organization of the information collected.
- Problems cannot be identified unless an assessment has been made first.

Goals

- Short- and long-term goals are set.

Care planning

Taking into account the environment, equipment available and nurse skill mix:

- A plan is formulated by the nurse, patient and family;
- The problems are dealt with in order of priority.

Nursing action

- The nurse and patient, where possible, carry out the plan.

Evaluation

- All action is examined to see if it has achieved the desired goal.
- If the goal has not been achieved the assessment process is recommenced.

Example: a patient with a head injury

Assessment

- Listen to what the patient is able to say/not say.
- Talk to the patient and family to find out how, when and why the injury occurred. Also, to find out more about the effects of the injury on them.
- Observe the patient for effects of the injury.
- Touch patient to establish any other effects.

Problem identification in order of priority

- Airway possibly at risk.
- Bleeding from laceration of the scalp.
- Possible pain.
- Worry and fear of patient and family.

Goals

- To maintain airway.
- To stop bleeding.
- To recognize and help reduce pain.
- To alleviate worry and fear in the patient and family.

Care planning

- Position patient to maintain patent airway, observe and report changes.

- Apply pressure to area of bleeding, observe.
- Observe for signs of pain and report changes.
- Provide patient and family with means of obtaining information relating to all events.

Nursing action

- All aspects of the care plan are performed and the patient and family are involved whenever possible.

Evaluation

- This is done as soon as possible, and the patient/the family involved whenever possible, and re-assessment done as necessary.

From these stages and the example given, the organization of care and series of events can be seen.

People using the A and E department are individuals as well as belonging to social groups such as the family. This should be considered when using the nursing process. Many factors, such as the environment, equipment and the skill mix of nurses in the department, will affect its usage and importance must be placed on these variables if it is to work in practice.

The nursing process is:
Thinking-awareness-assessment-thinking-action-evaluation-assessment and this leads to *needs of the patient and family/significant others being identified and appropriate action taken.*

PROBLEM IDENTIFICATION – IS THIS A PROBLEM FOR NURSES?

In order to find solutions to nursing problems, it is important to identify what is causing the patient and family problems. Bower (1982) states that 'the largest part of the solution of the problem lies in knowing what you are trying to do'.

Example: a patient arrives in A and E following injury to his leg

- What are the nursing problems?

The leg injury is *not* a nursing problem, it is the *effects* of the *injury* on the patient and family that provide nursing problems. These can be described as nursing/patient/family problems.

A knowledge of the mechanism of the injury and the physiological effects on the patient are important, but problem identification does not end here. There are also the psychological, social, spiritual and cultural effects to be considered.

• How do the patient and family perceive their problems?

To continue with the same example, the nurse may identify the following problems: inability to move limb; pain; worry.

If consulted, the patient may identify the following problems: worry; fear; pain; inability to move.

What is shown here is the different emphasis that could be placed on similar problems identified by the nurse and patient. It is essential, therefore, that nurses take the opportunity, whenever possible, to discuss problem identification with patients and identify the importance placed on a particular problem and the reasons for this. Failure to do this could increase the worry and fear experienced by the patient and his family. Owing to the nature of the work in A and E, it is accepted that this course of action may not always be possible. However, this should be the aim whenever the situation allows.

As a result of discussion between the patient, nurse and family the following problems may have been identified:

• Possible loss of circulation: *physical*;
• Pain: *physical*;
• Concern about informing work, other family members and other commitments: *psychological*;
• Concern for the immediate future and long-term effects of injury: *social and cultural*;
  Some problems such as pain are also of concern to medical staff and can be described as nursing, doctor, patient and family problems.

DOCUMENTATION

This is seen as an essential part of the nursing process but seems to cause the most problems to nurses.

Advantages

- Documentation is a *record* of nurses' problem identification, action and care.
- It shows the effect of care and what happened afterwards.
- It provides evidence of continuity of care from the initial assessment to final outcome.
- It is a legal record.
- In addition, documentation provides information for research and education.
- Also, it is an informative record should the patient be re-admitted to A and E.

Therefore, it is a means of communication which would be useful at busy times when things can be forgotten or misunderstood. Also, it gives an indication about the role of the nurse.

Documentation can additionally be used to provide the means to collect evidence: for example, to support arguments that more nurses and equipment are needed. However, it is important that the nurse is aware of what constitutes nursing action.

Perceived disadvantages

There are a number of perceived disadvantages to the use of documentation. These include:

- It is time consuming;
- Uncertainty about what to write;
- In some cases, the written work is done after the care is given;
- Sometimes, the information is written down and then not acted upon.

It is important, therefore, to examine whether this is the fault of the nurse or the fault of the document design.

In the USA, two methods of documentation are used: source orientated record keeping (SOR) and problem orientated medical records (POMR). Both types of documentation are discussed here as they generate much information recording in their present state but there is scope for adaption to suit the needs of various A and E departments. It should also be stated that many other methods providing guidance for documenting information are available. All methods should examined.

Source orientated record keeping (SOR)

This is the traditional method of recording information. Each professional group (source), nurses, doctors and others, keep a chronological record of collected information (data) about the patient in a separate area of the patient's notes. For example, one part of the records will be medical notes, one nursing notes and another part laboratory results.

Advantages

- There is access to each discipline.

Disadvantages

- Problems are hard to define as each admission has a separate entry of problems.
- Delays can occur as patient notes are sorted for a specific piece of information.
- Accuracy of information depends on who has recorded it and how much value they place on a particular piece of information.

Problem orientated medical records (POMR)

This type of documentation was developed by Dr Lawrence L.Weed of the University of Vermont, USA, and has the following characteristics:

- It is a birth to death problem list which is updated at each patient visit to the hospital;
- A problem solving approach is employed, in which all health care personnel can identify and document problems. This is followed by planning, delivering and evaluation of care and treatment. Thus, it correlates with the stages of the nursing process.
- A central computer bank provides information about the patient at any time and anywhere.

It is made up of:
- Database/initial assessment by each professional group;
- Problem list;
- Initial plan;
- Progress notes;
- Discharge summary.

Database

- All health care personnel ask questions relevant to them. Nurses ask questions relating to nursing care, and doctors ask those relating to medical assessment and care.
- All collected information is recorded using the same database. This collected information will include:
  The chief complaint and reason for coming to the hospital;
  Personal and family history;
  Allergy and reactions;
  Medication.

Many of these questions are asked by medical staff during the patient's first visit to the hospital. They then remain on record and are updated as necessary at future visits. The nursing assessment (see nursing process and medical assessment) follows.

Problem list

These are cumulative lists of identified actual and potential problems requiring care and treatment. One list records nursing problems, one records medical problems and other lists may be available made up of problems identified by other health care personnel.

Example from nursing problem list:

Name . . .
Nursing problems identified . . .
No: 1
Problem: Pain
Date/time identified: 1/1/1989 at 0900
Date/time resolved: 1/1/1989 at 0910

No: 2
Problem: Cold house
Date/time identified: 1/1/1989 at 0900
Date/time resolved: 3/1/1989 at 1500

No: 3
Problem: Pain
Date/time identified: 4/6/1989 at 1000
Date/time resolved: 4/6/1989 at 1010

This then becomes a reference list for the nursing problems that are identified and additions are made at each patient visit to A and E. Similar ways of documenting patient problems could be used in more A and E departments, as patients returning to A and E would have readily available records of past solutions or actions. For example, an elderly person who has been treated in A and E and is ready to go home, may have on his records that he lives by himself. In which case, the problem list might state that there were problems with a cold house at the last visit. The problem was resolved and reference can be made to this.

Problems will be identified and indexed in the same way for all other health care personnel.

Initial nursing plan

This is similar to a care plan in the nursing process and includes patient education plans. There will be a plan for each health care personnel group. This then produces integrated notes for all disciplines.

Example from nursing care plan:

Problem	Goal	Plan
1. Pain	To relieve	Analgesia
		Other forms of pain relief

Progress notes

All health personnel use the same format of progress notes which are comprised of flow sheets and narrative notes in chronological order. Therefore, information can be found in nursing, medical and other health care personnel progress notes.

There is a specific format for progress notes which is known by all health care personnel as *soapier*.

Soapier
S–subjective data (what the patient states is felt).
O–objective data (what is observed/inspected).
A–assessment (on-going).
P–plan.
I–implementation of a plan.
E–evaluation of implemented plan.
R–revision of plan if ineffective.

Flow sheets record precise nursing actions at the time they are performed (e.g. observations of TPR (temperature, pulse and respiration) and BP (blood pressure), altering the position of the patient and giving an injection).

Narrative notes provide a summary of all care given. Problems in both flow sheets and narrative notes are referred to by their number and *soapier* letter.

Example of flow chart
1. Pain 1/1/1989. Analgesia given at 0905.

Example of narrative notes
PROBLEM: 1
DATE and TIME: 1/1/1989 at 0900

Notes: S I feel pain
        O pulse raised, sweating
        A patient has pain
        P analgesia, elevate leg, other forms of pain relief
        I analgesia given at 0905
        E pain relieved

Discharge summary

This is a resumé of the care received by the patient while in A and E, and it is made up of information supplied by nursing, medical and other health care personnel. Each identified problem is taken and a *soapier* note written. This provides a comprehensive report of all that has happened to the patient while in A and E.

Summary of example given
Name . . .
Nursing problems identified . . .
No: 1
Problem: Pain
Date/time identified: 1/1/1989 at 0900
Date/time resolved: 1/1/1989 at 0910

Initial nursing plan

Problem	Goal	Plan
1. Pain	To relieve	Analgesia Other forms of pain relief

Progress notes
Flow sheet
1. Pain 1/1/1989 analgesia given at 0905

Narrative notes

Problem	Date/time	Notes
1. Pain	1/1/1989 at 0900	S I feel pain O pulse raised, sweating A patient has pain P analgesia, elevate leg, other forms of pain relief

I analgesia given
at 0905

E pain relieved

Advantages to using POMR

- There is access to all data
- All problems are readily identified
- All health personnel can see others' contribution to care and treatment
- Problems are dealt with by all health care personnel and everyone contributes to its solution
- Useful for teaching and research

Disadvantages to using POMR in A and E

- Lack of time in which to write down large amounts of information
- Documents for recording information need to be designed carefully

It is important to note that care has to be of the problem solving kind before this approach can be used effectively. The nursing process and a model of nursing are needed.

Points for discussion:

- What kind of information should be recorded in A and E?
- How could problems of recording information be overcome?

Some of the issues surrounding the documentation of information will be discussed in chapters 5 and 6. However, it is important that the nurses in A and E departments work through their own ideas and find a form of documentation that works for them, something that enables them to record all care given to a patient and family. It may be that an adaptation of the *soapier* documentation, incorporating the stages of the nursing process and a nursing model, is appropriate. Alternatively it may be another method that is more suitable.

MODELS

A model is three dimensional reproduction usually on a smaller scale, a design (Oxford Mini Dictionary, 1984). Before beginning construction of a house, a model of the finished product can be built to illustrate the design. This would be a three dimensional reproduction of the house, built to a smaller scale. By examining this, potential customers could have a clearer idea of what they would be buying.

Some models can be dismantled and then re-assembled. The advantage of this is that the different parts can be seen and examined. The model house can have the roof removed and doors and windows taken out. Should the customer wish, these parts can be altered in the real house. If they prefer a window or door to be moved, instructions can be given before the house building starts, thus ensuring that plans and action can be reorganized. Without the model, the customer may not realize the relationship of doors and windows to other parts of the house until it is built, leading to disappointment that could have been prevented. Models, therefore, are useful. By representing reality they can help organize our thoughts.

A model, when linked to the house building process, can help identify and solve problems in the early stages of construction. Through the house building process, work can be organized, a plan devised and action taken. Reference to the model aids early problem identification. Professions use models: law, teaching, computing. These models are not constructed in a way that they can be touched and examined. They are constructed through words. In this way the model can be read and examined. To make understanding easier they are usually broken down into parts, each part complementing another; put the parts together and the whole is formed.

Professional models aim to demonstrate what a profession is and how it functions. Most are based on a philosophy; implicit or explicit. The philosophy is the foundation of the model, it influences the model's use within the profession and helps keep the parts connected.

The professional model can be applied to the jobs done by that profession, and is linked to a process of work: assessment, goal setting, planning, action and evaluation. This assists in the correct organization of work. Reference to the model at the start and throughout the job helps identify problems, and organized work helps solve these.

Nursing uses models in conjunction with the nursing process. Before these are introduced the medical model, familiar to many nurses, will be described.

THE MEDICAL MODEL

This model adopts a problem solving approach, and its underlying philosophy is that a person is made up of a collection of physiological systems. For all the systems to work in harmony a balance has to be maintained. Should one system start to malfunction, intervention is necessary to restore normal functioning. Failure of intervention leads to continued imbalance which can produce physical and psychological changes within the person.

In order to identify the problems, *assessment* is necessary. Talking, listening, examination and investigation of parts of the body lead to identification of physiological problems. Once the problems relating to an anatomical system have been identified, the *goal* is to change this dysfunction to normal functioning, thereby restoring balance. A *plan* of action is formulated, *interventions* are carried out based on this plan. *Evaluation* follows and places importance on the success of interventions to correct the physiological imbalance. If these fail, others are considered.

It is rare for a *patient centred* approach to be used in the medical model, and interventions are based upon what has worked before for a similar condition. The person using this model, the doctor, decides what is best and the patient does or does not receive the treatment. Very little responsibility remains with the patient, leading to few patient centred decisions.

The medical model uses a problem solving approach, but

is different to the nursing process and nursing models. The person receiving treatment and care is viewed differently. In other words, the philosophy of care is different. Should a group of A and E nurses' philosophy readily identify with that of the medical model, this one may be the one of choice for that particular department.

However, these question should be asked first:

- How do patients and their families perceive their care in A and E?
- Does the medical model offer a basis from which patient care can be planned and delivered?
- Does it take into consideration the value of the role of the A and E nurse?

NURSING MODELS

Nursing models represent nursing. They provide a definite way of collecting and organizing information. There are many available and most have an underlying philosophy which considers and clarifies the meaning of health, ill health, the individual and the role of the nurse. Roper, Logan and Tierney (1983) use activities of daily living to guide nurses into collecting information and organizing it. Orem (1980) uses self care principles and the Human Needs Model (Minshull *et al*, 1986) a hierarchy of needs approach. Each nursing model provides slightly different guidance depending upon the author's views of nursing and the individual.

Nursing models, like many other professional models, are constructed through the use of words. By reading them the models can be examined. Much is written on the subject and authors invite nurses to apply what is read to the clinical area and the patient. However, this is not easy. Few nurses have access to the original work of the author for it is often written in complex language. This persuades the reader to abandon the work at an early stage before the author's full interpretations have been discovered, and many nurses rely on the descriptions of specific models by other nurses. These can act as an introduction to the model, but it is important that the nurse analyzes the original work herself in order to make personal decisions about the suitability of different nursing models.

Research is used to explain how certain models work but this has to be put into practice by other nurses, and for this a knowledge base is needed.

For the model to be used it is divided into parts. Each part can be compared to a stage of the nursing process. There is an assessment, planning, action and evaluation stage within each nursing model. These parts provide the nurse with a clear means of collecting and organizing information. Decision-making, care delivery and evaluation should follow. Without a nursing model the nursing process can still be used to accumulate and arrange information. The difference may be that the individual nurse will determine what is important. This decision could be based on the nurse's views and beliefs of nursing, role and the patient. All nurses have an image of nursing, an internal view of what the individual needs and how these needs should be met. MacFarlane (1986) states that most nurses have a good idea of how nursing and the practice of nursing should be.

Making these internal models explicit may provide the basis from which a suitable model of nursing can be chosen. Most individual nurses can identify with some aspects of a nursing model, and concensus may be reached through thought and discussion.

By using a model all nurses working within its framework use the same guidelines. This creates the potential for uniformity and continuity of care. However, the choice of a nursing model still remains difficult. This can be exacerbated by a non-clinical nurse choosing a model and then not taking part in the introduction of its use. The nurse may have experienced its use in one area, but this does not mean that it will work elsewhere. Consultation and discussion between those nurses who will have to use it in practice should precede any other clinical application. During discussions, the origin of the model should be examined. Many nursing models originate from the USA, and this can present problems as these may contain different views and values relating to the role of the UK nurse as well as cultural differences.

Points for discussion:

- How can the use of a nursing model be applied to A and E nursing?

The application of nursing models to A and E nursing

A nursing model in A and E should be adaptable enough to deal with all nursing situations. A workman uses a selection of tools to accomplish a variety of jobs. So, an A and E nursing model should have a selection of workable elements within it as it is necessary to have flexibility for this type of nursing.

Some aspects of nursing model usage in A and E which should be considered include:

- The assumption that nursing models will not work in A and E;
- Nurses in A and E need to examine the concept of nursing models;
- Nursing models should be tested in A and E departments;
- Use of a nursing model in A and E would promote examination of the role of the A and E nurse;
- Use of a nursing model could make A and E nursing more informed;
- A and E nurses need to choose a method of care organization based on thought, knowledge, examination and supporting evidence.

Example: care of a wound of the foot using the human needs model of nursing

Assessment

- Information is collected about the mechanism of injury, position, type, age of wound. Also, information about the patient and family relevant to potential wound care.

Problem identification

There is bleeding, pain, worry and fear.

Goals

- Short-term: to arrest bleeding; alleviate pain; overcome worry and fear; to promote a healing environment for the wound.
- Long-term: to promote wound healing.

Care planning

- Consider the immediate environment and the equipment available (types of instruments, dressing packs and dressings available).
- Pressure will be applied to the foot and the area observed for further bleeding.
- Methods of pain relief will be discussed with the patient and family, and analgesia given if indicated.
- The wound will be dressed appropriately.
- Information about all events will be given and question asking promoted.

Nursing action

- Nursing plan carried out.

Evaluation

- Bleeding is arrested
- Pain alleviated
- Correct dressing applied
- Patient and family are aware of the reasons for all the nursing and medical action. Information has been given about all aspects of wound care and follow-up treatment and care.

This problem solving approach using a model of nursing can be applied to the same patient on subsequent visits to the A and E department. Each visit may unveil new problems which need identifying.

Documentation

This is discussed on pp. 55–61 and in chapters 5 and 6.

NURSING PHILOSOPHY AND NURSING MODELS

The choice of a nursing model should be determined by the nursing philosophy of nurses working in a particular clinical area. Therefore, in A and E departments the model should reflect the views of the nurses in that unit.

After choosing a model, it is possible that it will be necessary to make adaptations once it is introduced into the clinical area. This will lead to development of the chosen model, but problems will occur if the chosen model is not based on an explicit nursing philosophy.

Most nurses have a good if not clear idea about the nature of nursing. Discussion will develop ideas and promote the formation of an explicit nursing philosophy. The importance of philosophy has been discussed (chapter 3), and once nurses have spoken about their ideas and how they see A and E nursing then there is a starting point from which to proceed.

In the following chapters the work of one group of nurses to find a suitable model for A and E will be introduced. At the beginning of this work, a group philosophy had not been made explicit. However, as the initial work progressed, nurses attempted to give reasons for preferring a particular nursing model, and it soon became obvious that attempts were being made to explain individual views of A and E nursing. Discarded models could not be readily identified with the views and values that determined how A and E nursing was performed. This influenced the formulation of a nursing philosophy. Nurses could then understand why one nursing model was chosen and the others discarded. The chosen one was readily identified with A and E nursing.

CONCLUSION

This chapter has covered many concepts. The reason for providing this information is to promote development of nursing models in A and E departments. Development will only take place once A and E nurses have decided what is suitable for them, and their choice should be based on knowledge, concensus and supporting evidence.

A nursing model should work in practice, and it should

provide a means of identifying problems relating to patient care in A and E. This then provides the basis for care planning, action and evaluation. This chapter concludes with two descriptions of the same nursing situation found in A and E.

Examples of nursing approaches in A and E

The following is a situation that could be found in A and E. Two examples of a nursing approach to this situation will be given to help demonstrate the use of a nursing model.

Mr Ronald Smith arrives in the A and E department accompanied by his wife Mary and son George. Mr Smith has been working in the cellar at home and knocked his right lower leg with a plank of wood. He has no other injuries.

Since injuring his leg, he has been able to walk a few painful steps. He is now complaining that he can feel a lump where the wood hit him. He is sitting in a wheelchair in the A and E department waiting room when the nurse meets him.

There are several ways in which Mr Smith could receive nursing care in A and E. Here are two examples.

Example 1

Nurse (N): Mr Smith?
Patient (P): Yes.
N: (to patient and family) Hello I'm ... Is this your wife and son?
P: That's right (family smile in acknowledgement), Mary and George.
N: (to patient) Right, I'm going to take you to a cubicle and look at your leg. Can your family wait here?

The nurse takes the patient into a cubicle, the family remain in the waiting room.

N: Okay you've hurt your leg? Which one?
P: The right one and it really hurts.
N: (who notices that the patient looks pale) First, I want to lie you down on this trolley.

The patient lies down.

N: How do you feel now?
P: Awful.
N: Can you get undressed?
P: Why?
N: So that I can see if you've hurt yourself anywhere else.
P: (as he gets undressed) I've only hurt my leg, nowhere else.

The patient continues to undress, the nurse can see no other injuries.

N: Right, how does your leg feel now?
P: It hurts.
N: Can you feel your toes?
P: Yes.

The nurse feels the toes and skin of Mr Smith's right leg and foot.

N: Good. Let me know if you can't. Right, the doctor will see you soon.

The nurse starts to leave the cubicle.

P: Can I see my family while I'm waiting?
N: Yes, I'll go and get them.

The family enter the cubicle. They all wait to see the doctor.

Example 2

Nurse (N): Mr Smith?
Patient (P): Yes.
N: (to patient and family) Hello, I'm . . . .. Is this your wife and family?
P: That's right (family smile in acknowledgement), Mary and George.
N: (to patient) Right, I'm going to take you into a cubicle and look at your leg. (to patient and family) Do your family want to come too?
P: If my wife can come with me and George (nods to son) can ring work for me; they don't know I'm here and they are expecting me at 1400 (he looks at his watch).

N: (to patient) When George has made his 'phone call do you want him to join you?

P: Yes.

N: (to George) When you have finished, wait here and I'll come back and show you where your dad is. Do you know where the telephones are?

G: Yes thanks, I'll see you here shortly.

The nurses takes Mr and Mrs Smith into a cubicle.

N: (to patient) You've gone pale, are you feeling alright?

P: I feel awful, I've just had a sudden pain shoot up my leg.

N: You may feel better if you lie down.

P: Yes I think I will.

The nurse and Mary help Mr Smith onto the trolley.

N: How do you feel now?

P: Better.

N: Have you hurt yourself anywhere else?

P: No.

M: No he didn't, I was there when he did it.

N: I will have to have a look at your leg, so you will have to remove your trousers.

P: Okay, Mary can you give me a hand? (Mary helps).

N: (looking at the patient's leg and foot) Your skin is okay; the colour is good.

P: (also looking) Yes it is.

N: Do you normally have any problems with the circulation in your leg and foot?

P: No.

N: Do you have any pins and needles or strange feelings in your leg, foot or toes at the moment?

P: No.

N: Do your toes feel cold?

P: (wiggling his toes) No my toes and feet feel fine. I just have a pain (he points to the place) here.

N: When do you get the pain?

P: When I try to move my leg.

N: What sort of pain is it?

P: A sharp, shooting pain.

N: (putting his leg on a pillow) Does this help?

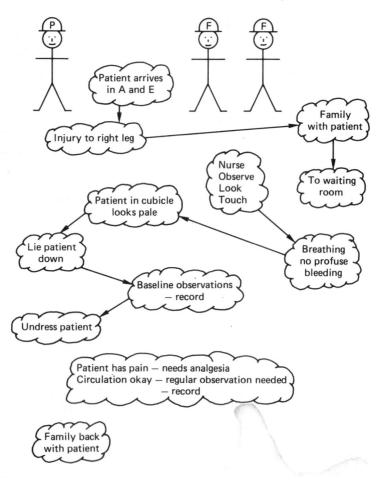

Figure 4.1 Summary of example 1.

P: Yes, it's more comfortable but the pain is still there (attempts to move his leg) ouch! When I try to move my leg.

M: Then don't move your leg.

N: I can't give you anything for the pain until the doctor has seen you, as she prescribes any pain killers that are needed. Can either of you suggest anything that may help reduce the pain in the meantime?

M: I'll talk to him and keep his mind off it.

P: Actually, I do feel much better than I did.

N: Let me know if your leg, foot or toes become cold, blue or white, or if you start to experience pins and needles or other strange sensations in these places. I will check regularly also.

M: Yes we will.

N: Will George have finished making the 'phone calls yet?

M: I'll go and check in a minute.

N: Okay, the doctor will see you as soon as possible. Do you want to know anything else? (Mary leaves and returns with George a few minutes later).

P and M: No, not at the moment.

N: Ask if you do, I'll return in 10 minutes and let you know how long you have to wait.

The nurse leaves.

Summary of example 1 (Figure 4.1)

- There is immediate removal of choice by the nurse contributing to loss of decision-making by the patient and family.
- The patient is isolated from the family; little reason is given for this by the nurse.
- Verbal cues from the patient are ignored by the nurse. Patient's answers have little effect on nursing actions, particularly in relation to pain and its effects on the patient.
- On several occasions the patient is expected to follow instructions with little information, for example lying down on the trolley, telling the nurse if he cannot feel his toes and waiting for the doctor.

Summary of example 2 (Figure 4.2 a and b)

- Throughout the meeting, the nurse acknowledges the importance of all family members by encouraging informed decisions to be made by them.
- The patient is seen as a person with a life outside the hospital. Value is placed on needs relating to other parts of the patient's life, for example the need to contact his employer.
- The nurse accepts the patient's decision to have his

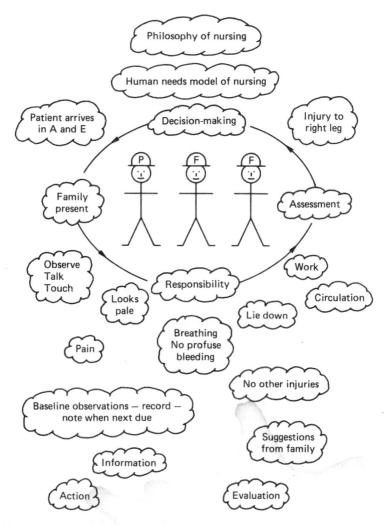

Figure 4.2(a)   Philosophy of nursing (human needs model of nursing).

wife accompany him to the cubicle and take part in his care.

1. In this example the nurse, patient and family identify the following problems:

- Possible problem with *circulation* in patient's right leg.

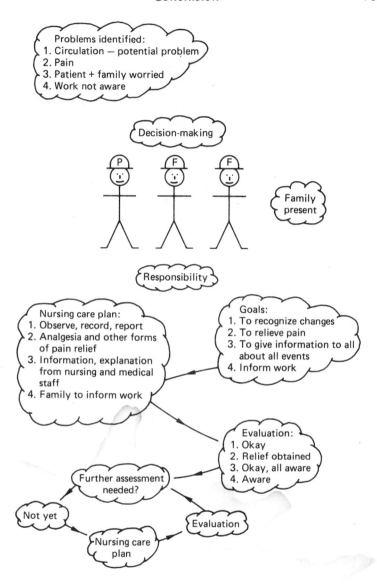

Figure 4.2(b) Summary of example 2.

- *Pain* in right leg.
- The *patient* and *family* are *worried*.
- The patient's *employer* is *not aware* of his arrival in A and E.

2. The following *plan of care* is formulated:

- Circulation: the nurse, patient and family will observe and report any changes. The nurse will record all findings.
- Pain: the nurse, patient and family will seek and provide reassurance and explanation. The right leg and foot will be elevated. Analgesia may be prescribed by the doctor.
- Patient and family are worried: information and explanation will be given by nursing and medical staff. Question asking from the patient and family will be encouraged and acted upon.
- Work not aware: the patient's son will inform patient's place of work about his visit to the hospital.

3. *Evaluation*:

- The circulation remains adequate.
- The pain is not yet relieved but the patient is more comfortable and is aware of the reasons for withholding analgesia.
- The family are less worried, they can see the patient is more comfortable. They are aware questions can be asked and that the nurse will return shortly.
- Mr Smith's employer is aware that he is in A and E and has given him time off until further notice.

4. *Documentation* (see chapters 5 and 6).
   This can be summarized as follows:

1. Problems identified

1. Circulation
2. Pain
3. Patient and family worried
4. Work not aware

2. Goals

1. To recognize changes
2. To relieve pain
3. To inform patient/family about all events
4. To inform work

3. Nursing care plan (stop – look – listen)

1. Observe, record, report normal condition and changes
2. Elevation, other pain relief and analgesia
3. Information/reasurrance from nursing and medical staff
4. Family to inform work

4. Evaluation

1. Satisfactory
2. Relief not obtained but more comfortable
3. Everyone aware of events so far
4. Aware

5. Further assessment needed? No – continue with care plan – evaluation

In example 1, the nurse is concerned with the patient's injury and fails to see the importance of the effects this injury has on the person. The patient's physiological needs are inadequately met, and feelings of pain are ignored by the nurse. The nurse's behaviour is governed by the way patients with similar injuries have been dealt with before.

In example 2, a problem solving approach is employed. Needs in the patient and family are identified by involving them in the assessment. These needs are met through shared care planning and action.

Points for discussion:

- Which example describes and reflects nursing care found in A and E?
- If example 2 reflects care provided by some nurses, should steps be taken to share this approach with other nurses?
- If you were Mr Smith or a member of his family which example of nursing care would you choose?

REFERENCES

Bower, F.L. (1982) *The process of planning nursing care* (3rd ed.) (London: The CV Mosby Company).

MacFarlane, J. (1986) 'The value of models for care' in B. Kershaw and J. Salvage (1986) *Models for nursing* (Chichester: John Wiley & Sons).

Minshull, J., Ross, K. and Turner, J. (1986) 'The human needs model of nursing' *J. Adv. Nurs.*, vol. 11, pp. 643–9.
Orem, D.E. (1980) *Concepts of practice* (New York: McGraw Hill).
Oxford Mini Dictionary (1984) (Oxford: Clarendon Press).
Roper, N., Logan, W.W. and Tierney, A. (1983) *Using a model for nursing* (Edinburgh: Churchill Livingstone).
Wilson–Barnett, J. (1988) 'Nursing values: exploring the cliches,' *J. Adv. Nurs.*, vol. 13, pp. 790–6.

FURTHER READING

Kershaw, B. and Salvage, J. (1986) *Models for nursing* (Chichester: John Wiley and Sons).
Documenting patient care responsibily (1978) Nursing Skill Book Series (USA: Intermed Communications Inc).
McFarlane, J. and Castledine, G. (1982) *A guide to the practice of nursing using the nursing process* (London: The C V Mosby Company).
Pearson, A. and Vaughan, B. (1986) *Nursing models for practice* (London: Heinemann Nursing).
Wright, S. (1985) 'Real plans for real patients', *Nurs. Times*, August 21, vol 81, no. 34, pp 36–8.
Wright, S. (1985) 'A rich experience', *Nurs. Times*, September 4, vol 81, no. 36, pp. 38–9.

Chapter 5

Preparation for change

CONTENTS

INTRODUCTION

The process of change is the subject of this chapter, and a small selection of research projects in this area will be discussed. These will be linked to A and E nursing through the use of examples and discussion points. The application of the change process will then be examined and its relevance to practice will be discussed.

Four important components of an organization (task,

people, technology and structure) that are often subjected to the change process will be introduced at the beginning of this chapter. There will then be discussion about the problems which may occur as change is implemented, including resistance and varying attitudes.

The second part of the chapter links theory to the preparation for change as carried out by one A and E department. This will include descriptions of the involvement of the staff in the change process and discussion about the need for two-way communication which facilitates decision-making. The aim of this chapter is to provide information for discussion and a starting point from which those wishing to initiate change can develop their ideas, and emphasis is placed on linking change theories to practice. Thus, it is hoped that the application of such ideas will aid the development of nursing.

WHAT IS CHANGE?

Planning, preparation and progression through a series of events will determine the final outcome of the change process, (i.e. success or failure). It is important, therefore, to understand the meaning of change and its implications. According to the Oxford Mini Dictionary (1984) it is defined as 'make or become different'. This definition does not make the process of change any easier to describe. For, what the dictionary describes so explicitly in four words cannot match the effects such a concept has when applied to a situation, place or person.

For descriptive purposes, the word 'change' can be visualized as a number of boxes (Figure 5.1). Each box contains certain tools which, when used sufficiently, enable another box to be opened and used. All boxes should be used frequently and as the situation requires. This is only one way of visualizing the change process; there are others which will be discussed.

Change is usually a response to a perceived problem or need, and is executed in many ways; through task, structure, technology, people. Whatever the origin and no matter which of the four mentioned routes are taken, people, the job they do and the environment in which they work will all be touched by the change.

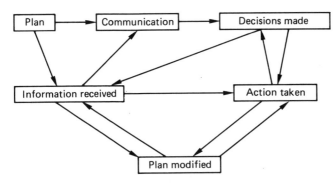

Figure 5.1 Visualization of the word 'change'.

In A and E departments such change is going to affect the nurses, the patients, other members of the multidisciplinary team, jobs done and the daily running of the department, the structure and methods used to solve problems.

Points for discussion:

- How would you define change?
- How would you explain your definition in visual terms?

THE ORGANIZATION WHERE CHANGE IS TO TAKE PLACE: THE A AND E DEPARTMENT

The A and E department can be described as an organization that is made up of, among other things, people interacting within groups. The department functions within another organization; the hospital. Therefore, changes within the hospital organization will affect the A and E department and vice versa.

There are many aspects of an A and E department that are subject to change. However, the emphasis in this section will be on task, people, structure and technology.

When change is initiated, it is usually with a view to modifying one of these components. However, as the change process progresses, other components become affected. It can be difficult, therefore, to establish which component was originally responsible for the change process, thus reinforcing the complex nature of the change process.

Points for discussion:

- Which parts (components) of the A and E department would you consider altering, thus initiating change?

THE FOUR COMPONENTS INVOLVED IN THE CHANGE PROCESS

Task

This section covers work that is usually performed by individuals within the organization to create a product. This then enables the organization to function. For example, in a factory, tasks may be performed to produce toy cars. These then become a source of income enabling the organization to buy more raw materials to make more toy cars. Changing a particular task in response to a specific problem may be considered very important as a means of improving output and income in the factory.

In nursing, the *task* is often related to patient care and can be the basis for many change processes, the hypothesis being:

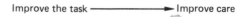

Improve the task ——————————▶ Improve care

For example, the task may be the taking of a temperature. Change may be initiated as the need to review the cleaning of thermometers is identified. This example can be summarized as follows:

- Task—Taking temperature;
- Perceived problem—Are thermometers cleaned enough?;
- Investigate—Need for change;
- Change initiated—Thermometers cleaned with solution x.

Another task may be the renewal of a patient's dressing. There may be a wish to implement change following new evidence related to the use of cleaning solutions.

Again, this example can be summarized as follows:

- Task—Renewing a patient's dressing;
- Perceived problem—Is the correct cleaning solution being used?;
- Investigate—Need for change;
- Change initiated—Solution y used to clean patient's wounds.

From these examples, it can be suggested that the events producing the change (problem identification, investigation, change initiation) should affect other parts of the organization. The most obvious effect will be on the people who are expected to adopt the changes in the task. This example does not show the involvement, feelings and attitudes to change that could be involved in such a process.

Points for discussion:

- How do you view the relationship between task alteration and nursing care in A and E?

People

These are the nurses, patients, families and others who are either receiving care or working in the department.

People are complex and work by Hovland *et al* (1953) highlighted the difficulties that can be experienced when attempting to fit people into the change process. Attitudes, lack of communication and resistance all affect a person's perception and response to change. It may be necessary, therefore, to introduce such factors as communication and involvement of people in order to facilitate change. This, then, will make the change process longer, as there will be more time being taken up considering the needs of people within the organization. However, lack of consideration of these factors can lead to failure to implement change.

Points for discussion:

- How would this method be used in your A and E department?

Structure

This includes many factors such as the nursing hierarchies in A and E and the hospital, and the routes of communication used: formal or informal; see pp. 103–105. It consists of the workflow, the skill mix of nurses, and the way work is coordinated and delegated within the A and E department.

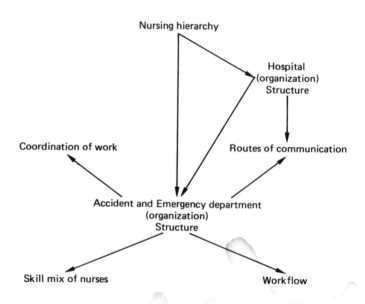

Example

Alterations in the A and E organizational structure may follow as more nurses are employed to work there. Such changes in the structure may affect the skill mix of nurses in the department, routes of communication, workflow and coordination of work.

Points for discussion:

● Discuss the ways in which increasing the number of nurses in A and E will affect its structure?

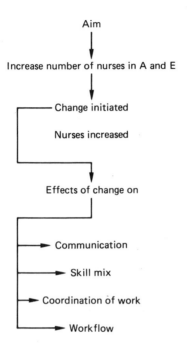

Aim

Increase number of nurses in A and E

Change initiated

Nurses increased

Effects of change on

- Communication
- Skill mix
- Coordination of work
- Workflow

Technology

This relates to the problem-solving methods used in A and E. The use of the nursing process and nursing models can be included here, as well as the problem-solving approaches used to find solutions to everyday problems and ways used to measure work. Change in these methods will affect the organization in many ways.

Technology also relates to equipment used in the department, such as cardiac monitors, ECG machines and, of course, computers.

Points for discussion:

- What specific problem-solving methods are used in A and E departments?
- How do these affect the delivery of patient care?

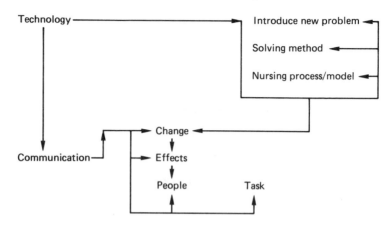

Change has been shown to take place in four main areas of the organization. Although the origins of change may lie in one of these four areas, a cascade effect is created as the change process is implemented. This may be planned for or be unexpected. The four components are only separated from each other here for descriptive purposes. Indeed, once the change process is in the advanced stages of planning or being implemented, they merge as they all become affected by this process.

Although change may be planned, no-one can account for the effects this change may have, particularly on people. Attitudes and resistance cannot be easily measured or anticipated in the planning of change. Outcomes relating to change may be acceptable or unacceptable.

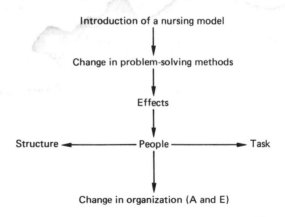

THE STRUCTURAL APPROACH TO CHANGE

This is the classic approach to change, based on deductive, logical and military thinking (Leavitt, 1964). The principle is that a well defined structure leads to optimal performance producing greater output.

This method focuses on solving problems, perceived as being present within the organization. Traditionally, the person perceiving the problem is in the organizational hierarchy at a management level, independent of the environment and those to be affected by the change. The change process, therefore, is not initiated by the people closest to the problem. No provision is made for change to be initiated by those individuals who are in the environment where change may be considered necessary. The person who is removed from the workforce observes the workforce and identifies a problem objectively, as an outsider. This process works on the assumption that by identifying solutions to problems and redefining jobs, output is improved and all objectives are achieved.

However, there are inherent problems with this method. Invariably, communication travels down the hierarchy to those who are identified as the individuals who must effect the changes, but at this point it ceases. This is often followed by the implementation of change as directed, with no allowance for time to be spent on reflection and communication.

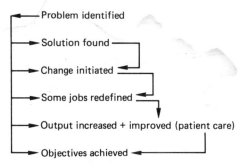

A nursing example of the structural approach to change could be the alteration of working hours. The aim could be to increase the number of nurses working in the A and E department at certain times during the day. This change may have been in response to information received, which identified a problem relating to the times nurses started and finished work. Communication would follow but little time would be available for reflection and response from those working within the environment (A and E) to be subjected to the change. This could have important implications as the alteration of working hours indirectly redefines the jobs of these nurses and such changes in the structure will affect how jobs are done.

Points for discussion:

- Would you expect there to be problems within the A and E department following this change?
- If so, what would they be?
- What factors have not been taken into consideration?
- Would improved output/patient care be achieved?

In effect, the structural approach to change looks at the task first and then makes decisions about the nature of the problem. After this, analysis continues backwards through divisions of labour up the hierarchy to identify further problems followed by rapid solutions (Figure 5.2).

The aim, with this approach, is to clarify and redefine people's jobs, especially those that have an end product.

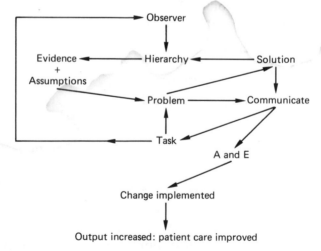

Figure 5.2   The structural approach to change.

The assumption behind this is that task performance will be improved. This method has been criticized as being formal, legalistic and based on little research evidence (Vroom, 1981). However, it is still widely used.

The structural approach to change makes assumptions about human behaviour; those having a contract will follow it and those given responsibility will accept it. Also, it is assumed that people will accept change and strive to meet identified goals set for them without question. There is no room for individual development in this process and no development of the work environment by those who work in it.

The problem perceived by the independent observer may not be seen as a problem to the individuals working within a particular environment. Indeed, the change process may produce more problems for the workers, and none of these factors seem to be taken into consideration. However, it is a quick way of implementing change and is done for the good of the whole organization. Once the problem has been identified, the process can be communicated and implemented without delay. Also, a problem can be identified objectively away from the work area where it is likely that subjective thoughts could affect a much needed change.

Points for discussion:

- Could this process be successfully applied to the A and E department where you work?
- What other advantages can you relate to this method of change?
- How successful would you consider this method of change to be in the long term?
- How important is the time factor in relation to the change process?
- Should individual needs be considered when implementing change?
- If so, what effect can this have on the change process?
- Discuss the ways that the following factors influence this type of change process:
  - Resistance of individuals to change;
  - Perceived loss of value by the individual due to changes in the job previously done;

- Position in organization and how the worker may see this being affected;
- Job satisfaction;
- Loss of social contacts within the organization.

This approach has been subject to modification (Chapple and Sayles, 1961). They criticized earlier work for failing to take into account human social variables when using this approach. They suggested, based on their work using applied social anthropology, that if the behaviour of people could be modified the task could be improved. Change would ultimately occur through the modification of workflow (structure) as already described but would take into account social groups at work and not just rely on altering people's work methods.

THE TECHNOLOGICAL APPROACH TO CHANGE

Traditionally, this type of change also focuses on problem-solving. It began earlier this century with the work of Taylor (1947) and has been used to alter structure, people and the way tasks are done. During its lifetime it has produced conflict as it has failed to take into account the emotional response that most humans have to change: block and resistance. Today, with the invention of computers this type of change is referred to as Operations Research. Some people may believe that this type of change and the movement towards more machines is for the better.

Both approaches to change have a body of technical methods for solving problems. Traditionally, both use external specialists to initiate change. This separates the specific planning of problem-solving methods, particularly in relation to the installation and use of machines (responsibility of external specialist), from searches for solutions to everyday problems (individuals in work environment).

Points for discussion:

- How could external specialists be helped to understand the way an A and E department functions?

In A and E there are many approaches to solving problems:

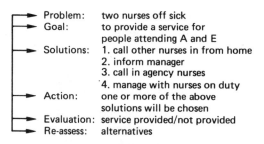

This is an example of a problem-solving method used by a nurse in charge of an A and E department.

A problem-solving method involving the change process would be the introduction of the nursing process and nursing model into an A and E department.

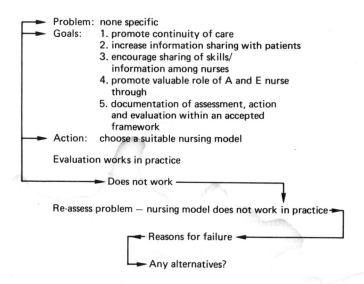

As already mentioned, this method of introducing change will eventually affect other parts of the organization (A and E).

Points for discussion:

• Is this method of initiating change suitable for A and E nursing?

- How much communication between members of the A and E department is needed for this method to be effective?

THE PEOPLE APPROACH TO CHANGE

This method suggests that aspects of an organization can be altered by modifying the behaviour of the people who work in it (Bennis, Benne and Chin, 1961; Ginsberg and Reilly, 1957).

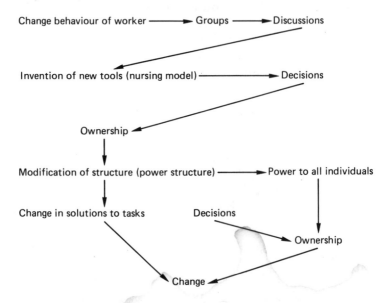

In the structural and technological approaches to change, the emphasis is on the need to solve problems. In this approach, however, there is greater attention given to the *whole* process of change and what this means to the people involved.

Historically, this process has moved through two phases. The first, the *manipulative phase*, looks at change as getting others to do what you want them to do (Carnigie, 1936). Carnigie focused on the relationship between the changer and the changee. Feelings and attitudes in the changee would need to be altered towards the changer and proposed change before behaviour changed voluntarily and could be displayed publicly. Carnigie promoted warm relationships with others and then bargained with them. This face-to-face influence has been supported by Hovland *et al* (1953), whose work included experiments on influence and persuasion.

The second phase has been called the *classical people approach* and deals with overcoming resistance to change. However, this approach still deals with the problem of finding ways of getting others to do what the changer wants them to do (Lewin, 1952; Cole and French, 1948).

Lewin (1952) and Cole and French (1948) were more concerned with increasing relationships among changees. By doing this, group pressure would occur. The effects of group pressure on individuals in the group would eventually bring about change. A key variable identified through this work was that of power and its effects on individuals and on the change process. Further work, therefore, attempted to remove the power variable. By introducing power equalization, ownership of the change and its results could be produced.

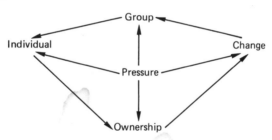

Rogers (1942) looked at client centred therapy, and Miles (1959) looked at group dynamics. Both looked at giving the changee at least equal power to those introducing the change. Training groups (T groups) developed and were aimed at teaching people how to lead and change groups and promote organizational change. T groups thus became the tool to promote change.

Bennis *et al* (1961) saw power equalization as an important aspect of change, as this provides the changee with the opportunity to influence change and retain responsibility for it. Group pressure can be created and promoted as part of the change process. However, support is needed from other group members if all the individuals involved

are to feel free to express thoughts, ideas and to make
decisions. Such group involvement in the change process also produces cohesiveness and conformity within
the group promoting ownership of change, an infusion of
new ideas and development of them. Communication is very
important for this process to remain successful. The more
channels of communication the better. This increases valid-
ity of information and individual commitment (see p. 103:
communication).

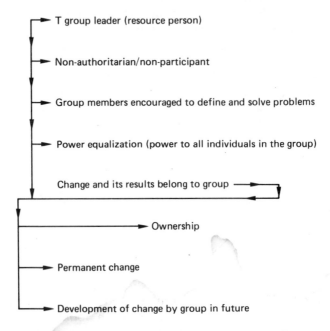

Points for discussion:

- How can this method be adopted for A and E?
- Do you predict any problems with using this method?

With relation to the types of change introduced:

- Which method would you consider using to initiate
  change in A and E?
- With which method would your colleagues, as the receiv-
  ers of change, prefer to be involved?

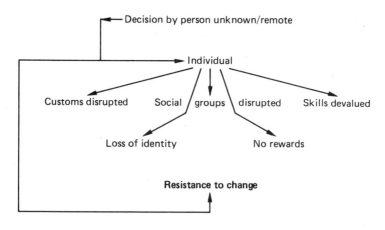

Figure 5.3 Resistance to change.

RESISTANCE TO CHANGE

When using any of the approaches described, there is likely to be widespread resistance to change (Graham, 1986). Possible reasons for resistance include the following:

- Decisions are made by a person unknown or remote from the individual and these have an effect on that individual and on the job that is done;
- Skills may suddenly become valueless through change;
- New methods relating to the delivery of nursing care can challenge the traditional role of the nurse. In addition, customs and rituals may be subjected to alteration;
- New relationships may have to be established. Change may involve the dissolving and reforming of established social relationships among nursing staff resulting in loss of familiarity and uncertainty;
- Resistance will occur unless some benefit can be seen, for example the opportunity to become involved in decision-making during the change process. Initially, any change involves time and effort on the part of all individuals. This can be seen as unbeneficial and inconvenient to the individual.
- Individuals generally resent being directly manipulated

by others within the organization. They can accept that some change will occur as a result of the senior– subordinate relationships in the hierarchy, but if more control than is usual is applied then resistance will result (Figure 5.3).

Points for discussion:

- How can these principles be applied to proposed change in the A and E department?
- How many of the above have you/your colleagues experienced?

ATTITUDES AND THEIR RELATIONSHIP TO CHANGE

Attitudes are comprised of three parts:

1. Cognitive (belief);
2. Effective (feelings);
3. Motor (a tendency to action).

Attitudes are an individual's characteristic way of responding to an object or situation, and are based on experience. A person learns to display certain types of behaviour or express specific opinions in response to a situation or object (Graham, 1986). They provide a predetermined set of responses and a person's behaviour and opinions can be forecast in certain situations. For example, an individual who has negative views about nursing models might display the following attitude:

- Belief—they do not work;
- Feeling—anger and resentment;
- Action—resistance leading to the nursing model not being used.

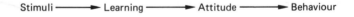
Stimuli ⟶ Learning ⟶ Attitude ⟶ Behaviour

Perception is strongly influenced by attitudes, and attitudes towards change will strongly influence reactions to it.

Altering attitudes

How can attitudes be altered?

- It is necessary to establish a group first, as the changing of attitudes occurs through exposure to group dynamics.
- Through exposure to the feelings, ideas and actions of the group, pressure may be exerted on the individual to make her conform to group standards. This is particularly true if the individual wishes to belong to a specific group (for example, nurses in an A and E department). By conforming to group standards, the individual will eventually have to accept group attitudes.
- The group exposes the individual to the attitudes of its members through discussion and the acting out of real or imaginary situations.
- Changes can occur through highly respected individuals in the group. Individuals model their words and actions on the respected person, sometimes without being aware that this is being done.

OVERCOMING RESISTANCE TO CHANGE

To help overcome prejudicial attitudes, so that change can take place, the Force Field Analysis (Lewin and Cartwright, 1951) can be consulted. This theory includes the following points:

- The factors that are producing resistance (environmental, people and objects) need to be identified;
- Once identified, it is necessary to determine the strength of resistance;
- Measures, such as better communication and information-giving, should then be introduced to overcome the resistance as soon as possible;
- Time is then needed for individual reflection about the information received. This should be followed by discussion and examination of ideas;
- Overall, this should result in a positive change in attitudes, which is described as the *unfreezing* stage (Lewin *et al*, 1951);
- The following stages of *changing* and *refreezing* would then need to be passed through before the individual would feel comfortable and accept the change as part of their working lives;

- Time would be an important factor in this process;
- Communication and the exchange of information would continue through all the stages (Figure 5.4).

The ways in which the psychological and sociological dimensions of a situation can affect the result are shown in Figure 5.5 (Roethlisberger, 1941). According to this theory:

- Individuals interpret a situation that involves change

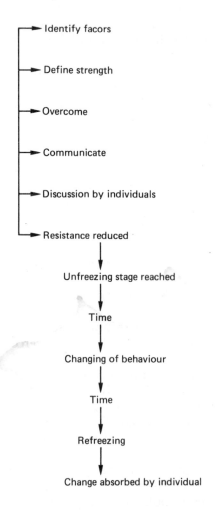

Figure 5.4 Overcoming resistance to change.

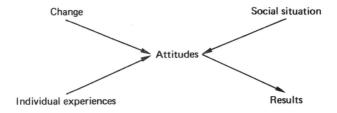

Figure 5.5 Roethlisberger's X chart.

according to their attitude to it. As stated earlier, attitudes reflect previous experiences and should be considered during the planning stages of the change process;

- During the change process, resistance will occur and should be recognized. It may be reduced with some careful planning prior to the introduction of the change process;
- All those who are affected by the change need to be informed as early as possible about the proposed changes and their method of introduction;
- People should be informed individually where possible;
- It is necessary to have individual participation in decision-making. If a decision cannot be made then as much consultation as possible should be used;
- Two-way communication is the most effective;
- Information will then allow the individual to re-assess her position in the new organization and look at the full effects of change. If necessary, she can then go back to the changer and clarify this;
- Information is also useful as the individual comes to reassess her value within the organization. Teaching can be offered here if new skills or approaches are needed;
- If possible, existing social groups should be preserved as they provide familiarity, stability and support for individuals while the change process is being undertaken;
- An understanding of the effects of change on others should also be shown, no matter how small the group, through regular contact with the changer.

IMPLEMENTING CHANGE

It is usual for individuals and groups to react psychologically to change. In other words, the response is normally emotional, and persuasion and rational argument may not be accepted. The following points are closely related to overcoming resistance to change (see pp. 97–99) and should be considered when implementing it:

- The changer should be viewed as an expert by the changees. This validates the whole process for those individuals taking part;
- The facts of the situation should be given to all involved individuals as soon as possible;
- Individuals who are held in esteem by the group should be chosen to take an active part in the change process. Acceptance of change should then occur in the group through them;
- Individuals should be allowed to take part in the stages of change and to adapt the final part for themselves. An active part in planning leads to *ownership*;
- Credit should be given to the workforce. It is necessary to be prepared to accept any small amount of change and to regard any movement towards the final goal as a positive step;
- It is important to be prepared for the change process to take longer than expected and to compromise on some aspects;
- Any change is a basis for future development.

According to Glen (1975) those people who actively support change are likely to be in the minority. The majority see change as providing some disruption and unsettlement in their lives. He sees change as a modification of a person's attitudes, and believes that it is both the cognitive (thinking) and effective (feeling) parts which will then lead to changes in behaviour. Even when change is known and accepted to be a move for the better, staff within the organization (A and E) can easily revert back to old established behaviours at times.

Dissatisfaction with a particular system does not automatically mean that individuals are any more willing to change.

The unsatisfactory system is still part of their working lives. As a result of it social relationships and routines have been established, some of which will be highly valued by the individual. Change will disrupt these.

Socialization, within the old system, involved the individual accepting group attitudes, some of which were different to their own. After a period of time within this system, security with what is familiar is established. Change can only offer uncertainty, for change reproduces emotions of uncertainty, anxiety and insecurity.

In their studies on nurses, Barton *et al* (1961) and Glen (1971) found that age and seniority played a large part in the acceptance of change. The older and more senior the nurse the less likely they would criticize the system and the less willing to accept change.

Point for discussion:

• Would similar studies today show the same results?

Social dynamics are always affected by change, and people's feelings need to be taken into consideration. Failure to recognize and deal with affective factors, such as anxiety and insecurity, will result in resistance to the change process and possible failure of the change process to take place.

TWO PLANS FOR CHANGE

Plan 1

This plan of change is related to Schein's (1965) work. There are six stages:

1. The need for change should be recognized;
2. Relevant facts and information about the proposed change should be presented to those in the organization who are viewed as being able to act upon them;
3. Modification of the change process will occur as feedback is received from those individuals taking part in the process;
4. The plan of change is altered accordingly, and any undesirable effects of change are removed as the plan is implemented;

5. The idea is then sold to a wider audience;
6. Feeback is obtained from this audience relating to the effects of change.

This work has since been developed, and more recent work takes into consideration the reasons for possible success and failure of change. However, the basic idea and approach to change remains.

Plan 2

Lupton's Change Plan (1971) offered advice to managers and those involved in the change process:

1. Define problem;
2. Look at all the alternatives;
3. Explore the present social systems of the organization including the external links with other organizations (A and E to wards);
4. List all groups affected by all the alternatives;
5. Examine issues likely to be raised by these groups;
6. Assess reactions from groups and decide on acceptability of ideas received;
7. Look at economic factors and feasibility against social acceptability, and take the course that offers low cost and is the most adaptive;
8. Explore problems raised by this course of action and attempt to deal with these.

Lupton recognized that even the best planned change can produce disruptive effects in the initial stages. These should be anticipated, accepted and dealt with appropriately as they occur. Adaptation of original ideas may be necessary as plans will be different once they are put into practice. The changer needs to be aware that, although the original idea might be theirs, the end result should be a mixture of ideas from those who have worked within the change process and those who have put forward suggestions for modification, producing ownership of the original ideas and future developments. Adaptation and modification of original ideas should occur as the change process and original idea develops.

Change should be planned in stages so that all of the

individuals involved can get used to the process and become involved. Acceptance is more likely if this course of action is taken. New ideas can be accepted gradually and become absorbed into the work patterns of those involved. Too much speed will increase resistance.

COMMUNICATION

According to Graham (1986), communication involves all processes by which information is transmitted and received. The subject matter may include attitudes and intentions, but the chief purpose of communication is to make the receiver of it understand what is in the mind of the sender. Messages must be received and understood for communication to be complete.

A result of understanding a piece of communication can lead to a change in behaviour. Therefore, effective communication is part of the learning and change process. Additionally, communication links an individual to others within a group or organization. For this reason, the form that communication takes is also important because it affects the receiver's attitude to the person communicating with them. Failure to understand what is being communicated leads to misunderstanding and possible distrust.

Points for discussion:

- How effective is communication in your department?
- Has change failed in the past because of ineffective communication?
- As a changer, with whom do you consider communication should take place in the department?
- How can you increase the chances of another person receiving your message correctly?

TYPES OF COMMUNICATION

Formal

Formal communication involves the written or spoken word and is planned or official. Usually, it is arranged and approved by those who are not working in the environment for which it is destined. Also, it is generally considered to be a more complete and permanent form of communication than those of informal methods. It could be thought that formal communication preserves authority and is a one-way process, as no provision is made for reflection and comment from the receiver, and there is often no upward flow of communication and decision-making by individuals at junior levels of the hierarchy. However, it is a quick way of getting a message across. Those sending the message may feel that this form of communication is appropriate.

Examples of this type of communication are:

- Letters;
- Announcements by notices;
- Memoranda;
- Large meetings addressed by a senior manager; communication remains one way as most people are inhibited by the seniority of the manager and the large numbers of people who are usually present. This method of communication is made permanent by the taking of minutes.

Informal

This type of communication is unofficial and unplanned. It is two-way and provides for reflection and a response from the receiver, thereby increasing participation in the decision-making process. It can be more time-consuming than formal methods as messages are received, considered and then answered. This extra amount of time should be incorporated into the plan of change.

Examples of this type of communication are:

- Small meetings;
- Interviews;
- Individual chats.

This type of communication demands patience and personal skills for it can be unpredictable. The sender may need to motivate the receiver to understand the message. The person using this method of communication within the change process needs to be adaptable and ready to accept ideas different from their own. However, decisions arising from such communication will be accepted much more readily.

Points for discussion:

- How important is the use of words, emphasis on words, speed of speech when communicating with someone?
- How accurate do you consider the following sentence to be? 'Often the intentions of the sender are not understood by the receiver because the sender is unsure of the message he/she is trying to send'.

PREPARATION FOR CHANGE IN ONE A AND E DEPARTMENT: INVOLVEMENT OF STAFF

Now that various theories relating to the change process have been described, the preparation for the introduction of change into an A and E department will be described. The change to be introduced was the implementation of a nursing model. The plan of change will be presented in chapter 6. If it is referred to here, it is only in relation to the involvement and information given to others within the A and E department.

The stages of preparation were as follows:

- It was very necessary to involve all staff from an early stage in this work;
- First, all members of staff were seen individually, as most people view any kind of change warily (see pp. 100–101) and anticipate some disruption to their working lives;
- The aims of the work were outlined and discussion took place as to why such work should be done. This gave each nurse the opportunity to make known her feelings in relation to the proposed work;
- Channels of communication were kept open and provided constant exchange of information;
- A brief resumé of each model was also made available to all staff. This promoted further spontaneous discussion and exchange of ideas;
- A written outline of the proposed work was given to each nurse. This included reasons for why and how the work was to be done, and details about the length of time it

would take and the ways in which it would be evaluated. The written outline would serve as a reference document, and as a guide to the stages of the proposed work;

- Most nurses, by this time, were well informed and were able to discuss views and ideas with others;
- Some resistance to the work had been anticipated and experienced. This was met with more information-giving and discussion, thus restricting the amount of resistance to a few individuals;
- Group discussions were also used throughout the preparation period;
- By the time the work began, all staff were willing to 'have a go'.

The aim of this preparation time, which began several weeks before the change was introduced, was to allow nurses time to explore all issues relating to such change. It was generally agreed that the introduction of a nursing model would not mean a great change in the way work was done. Many nurses in the A and E department were already able to demonstrate an ability to deliver planned care which had been systematically thought out. What was being introduced was a way common to all nurses that would provide the basis for assessment, action and evaluation. Those nurses able to demonstrate an ability to plan care systematically would now have the opportunity to share this with other staff. A framework (nursing model), which suited the needs of the department and reflected the shared systematic care planning and giving, would provide a common starting place from which further developments could take place.

The change was to be planned in small units, allowing all nurses time to absorb and to comment on events which were about to take place so that they could mould the work according to identified needs of the people in the A and E environment.

During the information-giving process the following were discussed:

- If at the end of the work it was proved that a nursing model was not suitable then other alternatives would need to be explored;
- From the work to be done, evidence would be collected

to support either the success or failure of the use of a nursing model in the A and E department;

- The final decision would rest with the nurses in the department;
- To remain with the old system (see pp. 80–81), evidence would still be needed to support the argument that this was the preferred method;
- The proposed work would involve time, work, effort and thought by all nursing staff as they were the ones who would work with the method eventually chosen.

REFERENCES

Bennis, W.G., Benne, K.D. and Chin R (eds) (1961) *The planning of change* (New York: Holt, Rinehart and Winston).

Barton, R., Elkes, A. and Glen, F.J. (1961) 'Unrestricted visiting in mental hospitals', *Lancet*, vol. i, pp. 1220–22.

Carnigie, D. (1936) *How to win friends and influence people* (New York: Simon and Schuster).

Chapple, E.D. and Sayles, L.R. (1961) *The measure of management* (London: Macmillan).

Cole, L. and French, J.R.P. (1948) 'Overcoming resistance to change', *Human Rel.*, vol. 1, pp. 512–32.

Ginsberg, E. and Reilly, E. (1957) *Effecting change in large organisations* (New York: Columbia United Press).

Glen, F.J. (1971) *Attitudes to change in the hospital service*: Paper presented at Occupational Psychology Section Conference (York: British Psychological Society).

Glen, F. (1975) *The social psychology of organisations* (London: Methuen and Company Ltd).

Graham, H.T. (1986) *Human resources management* (5th ed.) (London: Pitman Publishing Ltd).

Hovland, C., Janis, I. and Kelly, H. (1953) *Communication and persuasion* (New Haven, Conn.: Yale University Press).

Leavitt, H.J. (1964) 'Applied organisational change in industry: structural, technical and human approaches', in V.H. Vroom and E.L. Deci (1981) *Management and motivation* (Harmondsworth: Penguin).

Lewin, K. (1952) 'Group decision and social change', in G.E. Swanson, T. Newcomb and E. Hartley (eds) (1952) *Readings in social psychology* (2nd ed.) (New York: Holt, Rinehart and Winston).

Lewin, K. and Cartwright, N.D. (eds) (1951) *Field theory in social sciences* (New York: Harper and Row).

Lupton, T. (1971) *Management and the social sciences* (2nd ed.) (Harmondsworth: Penguin).

Miles, M.B. (1959) *Learning to work in groups* (Columbia: Bureau of publications, teachers college, Columbia University).

The *Oxford Mini Dictionary* (1984) (Oxford: The Clarendon Press).

Roethlisberger, J. (1941) *Manpower and morale* (Massachussetts: Harvard University Press).

Rogers, C.R. (1942) *Counselling and psychotherapy* (Boston, Mass.: Houghton Mifflin).

Schein, E.H. (1965) *Organisational psychology* (Englewood Cliffs, NJ: Prentice-Hall).

Taylor, F.W. (1947) *Scientific management* (New York: Harper and Row).

Vroom, V.H. and Deci, E.L. (1981) *Management and motivation* (Harmondsworth: Penguin).

FURTHER READING

Bennis, W.G. (1966) *Changing organisations* (New York: McGraw Hill).

Glanzer, M. and Glaser, R. (1961) 'Techniques for the study of group structure and behaviour', *Psych. Bull.*, vol. 58, pp. 1–27.

Proctor, T. (1982) *Management theory and principles*: M and E Handbooks (Plymouth: Macdonald and Evans).

Chapter 6

Implementing change: the introduction of a nursing model into one A and E department

CONTENTS

- Introduction
- The old system
- Problem identification
- Initial goals
- A plan for change
- Three models of nursing
- The action: a 12 week project
- Evaluation: results of the 12 weeks work
- The human needs model of nursing
- Further developments
- Advantages of using the human needs model of nursing
- Problems remaining
- The new system incorporating the old
- The new system versus the old
- References
- Further reading
- Appendixes

INTRODUCTION

The theories behind nursing model use (Chapters 3 and 4) and the process of change (Chapter 5) have been discussed in previous chapters. In this chapter, therefore, the aim is to describe the transition from nursing model theory into practice. This will be achieved by focusing on one A and E department. First, the 'old system' (use of nursing model documentation without a formal, accepted framework for care) will be discussed. This will be followed by specific points about goals, the change plan, action using three models of nursing and evaluation of the work done. Finally, the establishment of a new system, use of a nursing model in practice, will be described. It is hoped that this will lead to further work in this area.

Nursing models should develop as the environment and individuals change (Wright, 1986; Kershaw and Salvage, 1986). Such a concept is acknowledged in this chapter as nurses develop an understanding of the commitment they need to ensure the growth and evaluation of nursing models in practice (Wright, 1986). In this case, the human needs model of nursing was the one of choice and this is described. The advantages and problems remaining following adoption of the new system are then explored. Finally, the old and new systems are compared for similarities and differences.

THE OLD SYSTEM

The system used prior to the introduction of a nursing model consisted of individual nurses assessing patients based upon their own internal model of nursing; an awareness of this may or may not have been present (Kershaw and Salvage, 1986; Reilly, 1975). Action would then follow and the patient received care (Figure 6.1).

This was acceptable in many situations as the nurses giving care often had a wealth of A and E nursing experience and knew instinctively what the patient needed (Benner, 1982).

Points for discussion:

- Is it sufficient for a nurse to know instinctively what a patient needs?
- Does this concept of instinctive knowledge need exploring further?
- How is instinctive knowledge aquired and how can it be developed?

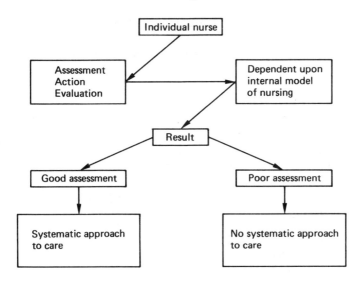

Figure 6.1 Old system based on internal model of nursing.

Documentation within the department consisted of nursing process sheets. These would be used for patients being admitted to the hospital only, the decision to admit the patient preceding the filling in of the nursing process sheet. Although the documents were known as nursing process sheets, the steps of the nursing process (assessment, action and evaluation) were not formally followed. The nurse completed the documents according to how she perceived the patient and family, their problems at that time and the environment. The amount of time available would influence the type and amount of information recorded.

The nature of the documentation process often reflected how long a nurse had worked in A and E, as experience gained while working in the specialty could influence the nurse's perception of the patient, family and all events surrounding them. This would be reflected in information recorded by the nurse. Some nurses would see the patient holistically, some did not. Again, this would be reflected in the type and amount of information recorded.

Information recorded was related to the patient and family, his treatment, nursing care and any other information considered important by the nurse at that time. Information relating to medical assessment, action and evaluation was also recorded by many nurses. This was a repetition of what had already been written by the doctor on the casualty card.

Points for discussion:

- Do you consider the documentation of nursing care in this way sufficient?
- What implications for care giving and receiving by nurses and patients does this method of documentation have?
- Should more nursing care be recorded?
- If so, in what way could this be done in a busy A and E department?

Some patient problems or worries may be omitted during the documentation process. This may be because they had not been identified or just not written down for whatever reason.

Points for discussion:

- Would the use of the nursing process with a nursing model overcome such problems?
- Would more problems be created for nursing staff if a nursing model were introduced?
- If so, describe these problems.

Some nurses in the department presented clear, accurate, concise accounts of nursing action and evaluation.

Points for discussion:

- Should these nurses be sharing their skills with other nurses?

Example of nursing in A and E using the old system

Two examples of nursing action are given.

The nurse's internal model (Kershaw and Salvage, 1986; Reilly 1975) enabled her to assess the needs of the patient quickly and to initiate action: nursing and medical. Once

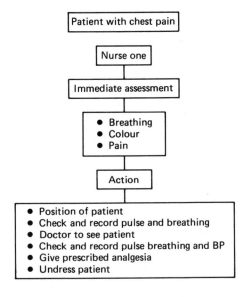

Patient with chest pain

Nurse one

Immediate assessment

- Breathing
- Colour
- Pain

Action

- Position of patient
- Check and record pulse and breathing
- Doctor to see patient
- Check and record pulse breathing and BP
- Give prescribed analgesia
- Undress patient

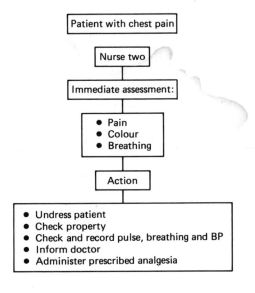

Patient with chest pain

Nurse two

Immediate assessment:

- Pain
- Colour
- Breathing

Action

- Undress patient
- Check property
- Check and record pulse, breathing and BP
- Inform doctor
- Administer prescribed analgesia

the patient is stable, the pain reduced, colour and breathing satisfactory then other needs can be assessed: social, psychological, cultural, spiritual.

The second nurse deals with the situation in a slightly different way.

She also works to an internal model of nursing, although this has resulted in different assessment and action.

Points for discussion:

- How would you account for the differences in assessment and subsequent action?
- Would a nursing model affect such differences in practice?
- What factors are likely to influence each of the nursing assessments?
- Discuss the possible outcomes for both these situations.

Another point considered was that of communication. Verbal communication was used extensively within the A and E department by all staff. No specific problems relating to communication had been perceived. However, general problems relating to communication were voiced by nursing staff intermittently.

Points for discussion:

- Describe the possible effects a nursing model may have on communication, both written and verbal.

From the description of the old system, it can be seen that many questions were raised relating to the non-usage of nursing assessment, action and evaluation and the whole concept of documenting nursing care. These are summarized here:

- There was no common framework for nurses to work within.
- Was it acceptable for an experienced A and E nurse to work by her own internal model of nursing?
- By providing a framework, experience used to assess patients and resulting priorities could be shared and used by all nurses.
- From a common nursing assessment, all nurses could plan care systematically. From this, evaluation would follow.

- Overall, this could contribute to the promotion of high standards of nursing care for all patients and their families attending the A and E department.

PROBLEM IDENTIFICATION

The problems with the old system were identified and it was found that there was no provision for assessment, planning of care or evaluation. Also, there was no formal use of the nursing process, even though nursing process sheets were available in the department.

No starting point for assessment of care

No provision for documenting nursing assessment

No provision for evaluating care systematically

No quick to fill in, easy to read nursing document

INITIAL GOALS

In trying to find a suitable model of care, the initial goals were identified as follows:

- The notion of nursing assessment with the events that should follow; action and evaluation would be explored;
- This would be done initially within the framework of a nursing model as yet to be identified.

Such a framework could incorporate the systematic approach to care already used by many nurses in the department. The overall aim was to reflect the vast range of skills available in the department. Such skills would be reorganized within a common framework of assessment, action and evaluation. Skilled nurses would then have the opportunity to share their experience with other nurses in the department, leading to a common distribution of skills.

- Continuity of patient care would also be explored. This would involve a nurse assuming responsibility for assessment, care delivery and evaluation of care to one patient. It was accepted that the nature of A and E work would not always make this possible but such a concept was not impossible.

- Information sharing with patients could be developed. Sharing information with patients through explanation and discussion should encourage them to take part in more decision-making relating to their care if they chose to do so.
- Methods of communication could be explored. Traditionally, A and E nurses pass on a lot of information verbally. The reliability of this information passage, especially when it involves passing this information on to others outside the department, was questioned.

At busy times and at handover periods should assessment, action and evaluation be documented, this might provide an extra route of communication, possibly reducing the chance of information being forgotten or misinterpreted.

A PLAN FOR CHANGE

Some principles of change have already been introduced (Chapter 5). However, for the purpose of this work, Lupton's change plan will be used and is reiterated here (Figure 6.2).

Define problem

The problem was defined that there was no framework available within which nurses could work to assess patients, and in which they could plan and evaluate care.

Look at all alternatives

In attempting to find alternatives to the old system, it was felt that there were no readily definable alternatives available that would provide a framework for a systematic approach to care.

Aims of the work

The aim of finding a new approach to care was to provide a means of promoting continuity in the care of patients and their families. It was also felt necessary to increase

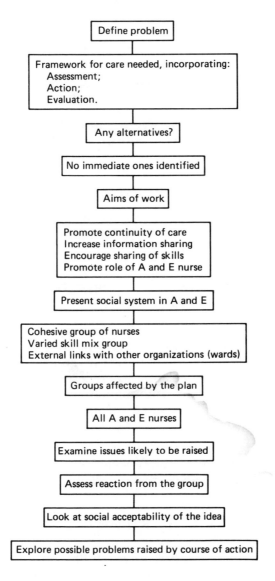

Figure 6.2 Lupton's plan for change.

information sharing among nurses, patients and others, leading to more patient/family involvement in care giving and receiving. Also, there was a desire to encourage sharing of knowledge and skills among all nurses in the department, and to promote the valuable role of the A and E nurse through the documentation of assessment, action and evaluation within an acceptable framework.

Explore present social system including external links with other organizations

It was found that a cohesive group of nurses existed in A and E. They worked closely with other health care personnel, patients and relatives.

Groups affected by the plan

The groups affected by the plan included all nurses in A and E, student nurses, visiting nurses to the department, patients and their relatives.

Examine issues likely to be raised by the group

The issues likely to be raised by the group that required investigation were as follows:

- Nursing models viewed as too time consuming;
- Not enough known about nursing models;
- Possible problems relating to the use of care plans;
- It was predicted that information and two-way communication would be needed to help alleviate anticipated issues.

Assess possible reaction from groups

It was felt that resistance was possible.

Look at social acceptability of idea to introduce a nursing model into the A and E department

There was positive social acceptability anticipated as the social groups were preserved, providing support and familiarity.

Explore possible problems raised by course of action

These included a need for more information and continuous discussion relating to nursing models and the planned work.

Outcome of plan

The following evolved from the plan.

1. Early introduction of a variety of information was needed, and it was felt that this should relate directly to the proposed work.
2. Interaction between individuals should be used to increase understanding about the work to be done.
3. Feedback from individuals would mould the development of the work.
4. Individual ideas should be incorporated into the change process as soon as possible enabling the plan to be altered as necessary. It was felt that by placing emphasis on the importance of involvement by individuals within the department the goal of ownership could be achieved.

After the formulation of a plan, the following statements were made known to all nurses about the use of a nursing model in A and E:

- It should provide a framework for assessment that could be utilized by nurses working in the A and E department;
- Following assessment the patient, family and nurse problems could be identified;
- Once problems had been identified, goals could be set and a plan of care formulated;
- Nursing action should follow;
- Care could then be evaluated.

Aim of plan

Any person (patient or relative) attending an A and E department in need of care has the right to a high standard of nursing care. The use of a nursing model and its subsequent documentation aims to provide this (Pearson, 1986; Castledine, 1986; Roper *et al*, 1985). In order to meet the initial defined goals of the proposed work, a cross-section of patients and families attending A and E would receive care within the framework of a nursing model.

A large proportion of the patients receiving care in this way would be those staying in the A and E department for a long period of time or those who had needs for which nursing action was required before they could leave the department. An example of the former would be a patient lying on a trolley following a leg injury; of the latter, an elderly person with a minor injury and identified social needs requiring nursing intervention prior to going home.

The reason for taking a cross-section of A and E patients in this way was to help integrate a nursing model into the department as smoothly as possible. Those patients who attended the department and remained in it for a short period of time would not, at this stage of the work, receive their care within the framework of a nursing model. For this may delay their departure from the department. Patients in this category would include those who attended the department, received treatment and left within a very short space of time. Documented nursing assessment, action and evaluation would not be required *unless* specific patient/family/nurse problems could be readily identified and acted upon. Examples of patients within this group whose care would be delivered within a formal framework have already been introduced.

Eventually, it was envisaged that the work would develop to include all patients and their families using the A and E department.

THREE MODELS OF NURSING

Following some discussion, it was proposed that three models of nursing should be introduced into the A and E department for a 12 week period. During this time, all previous nursing documentation would be discontinued. By using three models of nursing the nurses would have the opportunity to compare and contrast their use in the practical setting. Discussion could follow leading to one being chosen by the nursing staff working in the department that they felt suited the needs of the department.

There had already been an extensive literature search into the use of nursing models in A and E. Very little information had been found except reference to the use of Orem (Walsh, 1985) and an adapted form of Maslow (Frought and Trowe, 1984). Subsequently, the nursing models of Orem, Roper *et al* and the human needs model of nursing were chosen. Orem was chosen as it had been identified as being of use in A and E departments in this country (Walsh, 1985). Roper *et al* was also chosen as it was a nursing model familiar to most of the nurses in the department (Roper *et al*, 1983, 1985), and the human needs model (Minshull *et al*, 1986) as it represented a similar model to the one identified as being used in America (Frought and Trowe, 1984).

As three models of nursing were to be used, the permanent nurses in the department were divided into three groups, and each group worked with a particular model of nursing for a four week period. Each nurse received a brief resumé of the nursing model to be used in the first four weeks. This was followed by resumés of the other models as nurses worked with them. At the end of each four week period the effectiveness of each nursing model was evaluated using a questionnaire. This was completed by all nurses working in A and E at the time, including those nurses visiting A and E for a brief period, such as student nurses. After each four week period, the nurses then moved onto another nursing model, so that, at the end of 12 weeks, all nurses worked at some point with all three nursing models. It was suggested that students and other nurses working in the department for a short space of time follow the same model as their mentor. In this way discussion between the mentor and the student would take place about the value of the nursing model.

Following further discussion three nursing sheets were designed, one for each chosen nursing model. Each one incorporated nursing assessment as outlined by the authors' philosophy. For example, the documentation relating to Roper *et al* listed the activities of daily living as the main components of nursing assessment. It was also decided that nursing intervention would take the form of a written care plan followed by a written statement relating to evaluation.

A second sheet was then designed called the Biographical and Health Care Data Form. This was to be used to record all information about the patient and relatives, such as name and date of birth.

One point raised at this time was the ability of the nursing staff to formulate meaningful care plans in an often busy department. Concern was expressed about the time needed to write a care plan. After much thought and discussion it was decided to continue with the original idea to use care plans for the 12 week period to find out whether fears were founded or not. If they were, then evidence should be available to support the argument that the writing of care plans was unrealistic within a busy A and E department.

THE ACTION: A 12 WEEK PROJECT

The work commenced. All staff worked as had been directed and questionnaires were used to evaluate the effectiveness of the models in practice. It became clear very quickly that the human needs model of nursing would be the model of choice. However, the reason for this was unclear initially until work started on a philosophy of A and E nursing (Chapter 2). Once the beliefs and values held by the nurses in the A and E department were made explicit, the reasons for the choice of nursing model could be clarified.

EVALUATION: RESULTS OF THE 12 WEEKS' WORK

The following results were obtained after the initial 12 weeks' work.

- The A and E departmental philosophy could be easily placed within the human needs model of nursing. The model was sympathetic to the department's philosophy (Chapter 2). That is, it mirrored the views and beliefs of the nurses working in the department.

  It should be noted, however, that the nursing models of Roper *et al*, Orem or any other model of nursing may be suitable for other A and E departments. The choice of the human needs model of nursing for this particular department resulted from its ability to reflect and accommodate an already identified set of nursing beliefs. It is important that the philosophy does fit the model, as this should lead to realistic application of the model in practice (Wright, 1986).

- The chosen model would need modifying.
- The term 'nursing intervention' was misleading; nursing action would be used in all future documentation.
- Care plans were too time consuming. Patients often remained in A and E for a very short period of time, and it was felt that this period of time was necessary for immediate nursing care and that little time was available for writing care plans. This could not be said for all nursing situations in A and E, but was certainly seen as a problem during the 12 week period. Some other way would need to be found to document nursing action.
- Patients and their relatives stated that they liked being involved in care planning. They felt that it gave them the chance to ask the nurse responsible for their care other questions (this result was obtained by random, informal, verbal questioning of patients and their relatives by nurses).
- Similar nurse/patient/family problems were documented by all nurses for similar medically related and nursing problems.
- Some nurses felt that, in order to complete the assessment procedure accurately, it was necessary to do so much earlier following the patient's arrival in A and E (documentation was often left until it was known that the patient was to be admitted to a ward).
- It was difficult for some nurses to document what they did and not what medical staff did (this applied to all grades of nurses).
- Some nurses found difficulty in understanding that the assessment was for use in the A and E environment only and problems that might occur on the ward were not part of the A and E assessment process.
- It was sometimes difficult for the wards to understand what was being done. It was assumed by some wards that the A and E assessment should include identification of possible problems that may occur following admission onto the ward. Meetings and discussions between A and

E and ward nurses were used to try to overcome any problems.

These results indicated that the human needs model of nursing would be suitable with adaptation.

It was found that a method of documenting patient and family needs and problems was required. It was felt that this should be easy to understand, quick to fill in and read, accurate and that it should incorporate various types of information. Time and ongoing discussion would be necessary to develop this work further.

THE HUMAN NEEDS MODEL OF NURSING

The human needs model of nursing was originally devised to integrate nursing curricula, education and practice through the recognition of individual needs (Minshull *et al*, 1986). It was adapted from Maslow's (1954) work on motivation, and identifies five groups of needs: physical, safety and security, affiliation, dignity and self esteem and self actualization. These are placed within a hierarchy (Maslow, 1954), and are shown in Figure 6.3.

Within the framework of this model, it is recognized that any unmet need within the individual may lead to problems for the patient, nurse and family. Therefore, nursing assessment, action and evaluation, in partnership with the patient and family, identify needs and offer solutions to problems. This presents an holistic approach to care and embraces the philosophy formulated by the A and E department (Chapter 2).

Maslow's (1954) work proposed that an individual would only be motivated to meet needs at higher levels of the hierarchy once those at preceding levels had been met. The human needs model of nursing rejects this view. It acknowledges that certain physical, safety and security needs which are regarded as potentially life-threatening should be assessed first. Following this, equal emphasis is placed on each group of needs. This ensures that everything viewed as important to the patient, family and nurse is considered. Such an approach to individual needs is familiar to many A and E nurses.

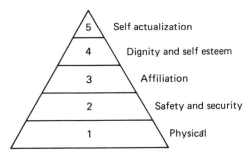

Figure 6.3 The human needs model of nursing (Maslow, 1954).

The life continuum within the human needs model ranges from the individual in maximum wellness to maximum illness. The individual is represented on the continuum as a triangle. Wellness is represented by an upright triangle showing the individual in a relatively stable state. On the illness side, the triangle is inverted and unstable. Support from the nurse is required if a stable state is to be achieved (Figure 6.4).

The nurse

The nurse has a supportive role within this model. In the illness state, the individual is assisted to recognize unmet needs through the assessment process. Problems are identified and care is planned, delivered and evaluated within a suitable environment. This should promote exploration of the implications of an altered health state by all parties.

In the wellness state the nurse's role is in the promotion of health and the prevention of illness/accidents. Nursing actions range from the provision of information to enable the individual to make more informed decisions to direct physical care.

Assessment

Assessing individual needs within the framework of the model provides a systematic approach to care allowing priorities to be established. Such an approach may reflect

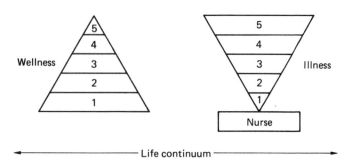

Figure 6.4 The life continuum with the human needs model of nursing. Reproduced with permission from Blackwell Scientific Publications Ltd.

the beliefs and values of A and E nurses. The nurse, patient and significant others can demonstrate that problems do or do not exist. Decisions relating to such problems can then be made by all involved parties. Only relevant information is sought, thus acknowledging the individual's right to privacy.

Intervention

This is achieved through partnership between the patient, nurse and significant others, when possible. However, it is accepted that, on occasions, the nurse may need to act independently if some goals are to be achieved, particularly in the physical needs category.

Evaluation

This is used to ensure that goals have been met. Failure to do so will result in reassessment.

The framework of the human needs model of nursing acknowledges the holistic nature of the individual. Such an acknowledgement may reflect the beliefs of A and E nurses.

FURTHER DEVELOPMENTS

After the preliminary study, other designs for the nursing document were suggested. The human needs model of nursing became the basic framework from which further ideas would generate. A number of attempts and considerable help were demanded from other members of the A and E staff. Finally, ideas were incorporated and a format accepted. The A and E nursing assessment, action and evaluation sheet then emerged (Figure 6.5).

The framework of this sheet is an adapted form of the human needs model of nursing. It incorporates biographical data questions which require a short answer. Therefore, nursing assessment and action have been placed together under headings of nurse/patient problems. The latter require a tick or short answer to show that they are present. Problems not present are not answered.

The ready documented problems are derived from re-occurring nurse/patient/family problems found during the original 12 weeks work.

The sheet covers physical, psychological and social problems which are of importance to the patient, nurse and relatives. Should any other assessment and action be identified, there is space on the document to record this. Finally, evaluation of care is done as necessary. The effects of medication can also be evaluated.

ADVANTAGES OF USING THE HUMAN NEEDS MODEL OF NURSING

It was found that the advantages of using the human needs model of nursing were as follows:

- The nursing assessment, action and evaluation sheet is a standardized assessment and action form. It is quick to fill in and easily understood by all involved in nursing care of patients and their relatives;
- The philosophy of nursing fits readily into the adapted model of nursing;
- Patients/relatives/significant others are involved in the assessment, care planning and evaluation when possible, and they seem to welcome this involvement. However, the type of nursing in the A and E department is sometimes of the 'doing for others' kind. Nursing action without patient/family involvement may be unavoidable at times. it is accepted that, in some situations, it is impossible to

**The A and E
nursing assessment, action and evaluation sheet**
(adapted from the human needs model of nursing)

Name: Presenting condition:
Prefers to be called:

Date/time of arrival in A and E: A and E no:

Address:

Telephone:

Date of birth: Religion:

Persons to be contacted:

Persons with patient in A and E:

Dependants (include pets):

GP address:

Support services:

Location of property/valuables:

Location of key:

Nursing measurements recorded: Frequency:

Please refer to charts/casualty card for all recordings:

Temp ( )   Pulse ( )   Resps ( )   BP ( )   Others ( )   specify _____

Cardiac monitor *in situ* ( )

The following nurse/patient problems have been identified:

1   2   3   4   5   6   7   8   please turn over

Figure 6.5 Nursing assessment, action and evaluation sheet.

1. Airway and breathing: Position of patient ( ) Suction ( ) Oral airway inserted ( ) Size ( ) O_2 given ( ) L/min, % ( ) Time commenced ( ) ET tube *in situ* ( ) Size ( )	**4. Pain** Area ( ) Type of pain ( ) Constant ( ) Not constant ( ) Analgesia given prior to arrival in A and E ( ) Time ( ) By whom ( )
2. Circulation: Limbs; identify ( ) Sensation present ( ) Movement ( ) Swelling ( ) Pulses ( ) Elevated ( ) Splint applied ( ) Rings removed ( )	Analgesia given in A and E ( ) Time ( ) **5. Body temperature:** Patient needs cooling ( ) warming ( ) Aids used ( )
3. Bleeding: Area ( ) Amount; Small ( ) Moderate ( ) Large ( ) Type ( ) Pressure applied ( )	**6. Fluid intake/output:** Oral fluids given ( ) Nil by mouth ( ) IV Cannula *in situ* ( ) Site satisfactory ( ) IV Fluids commenced ( ) Time ( ) Nausea ( ) Vomiting ( ) Diarrhoea ( )
7. Loss of familiar surroundings/ contact with others: Patient is aware where he/she is ( ) not aware ( ) Relatives contacted/aware patient is in A and E ( ) Not contacted/aware ( ) Reason ( ) Relatives are with patient ( ) Parents present ( ) Others present ( ) specify _____ Workplace contacted/aware patient is in A and E ( ) Not contacted/aware ( ) Reason ( )	**8. Freedom from fear** Necessity for physical examination; patient aware ( ) relatives aware ( ) Reasons for medical/ nursing procedures: explanation given to patient ( ) relatives ( ) by nursing staff ( ) medical staff ( ) Advice needed by patient ( ) relatives ( ) about this injury and further employment ( )

Describe any further nursing assessment/action taken:

Evaluation for 1 2 3 4 5 6 7 8:

Medication given as prescribed ( ) Time ( )
Effects of medication given _____

Patient's destination ( ) Patient aware ( ) Relatives aware ( )
Nursing sheet completed by _____ Time ( )

Figure 6.5 continued.

document nursing assessment and action until the patient has received the necessary nursing care and medical treatment;

- The nursing sheet has produced an extra route of communication that is directly related to patient care within the department. It is used as part of the nursing handover of patients and relatives within A and E, and from A and E to wards and other areas. It is becoming more widely read on the wards. Discussion with various wards shows that information documented by nurses in A and E helps the initial ward assessment.

PROBLEMS REMAINING

Confusion continued to arise when defining nursing action. A set of guidelines was made available to help nurses and discussion continued. Also, it was considered by some nursing staff that the nursing sheets were not filled in early enough following the patient's arrival in the A and E department. Discussion continued about this. Finally, feedback from the wards continued to demonstrate some confusion about the use of nursing documentation in A and E. This improved over a period of time.

THE NEW SYSTEM INCORPORATING THE OLD
Incorporation of the old system into the new system is illustrated in Figure 6.6.

NEW SYSTEM VERSUS THE OLD
A comparison of the new system and old system is shown in Figure 6.7.

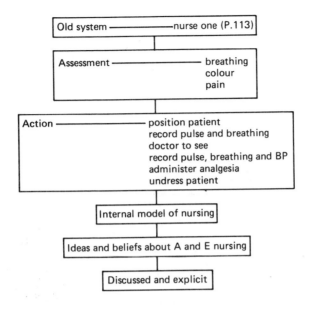

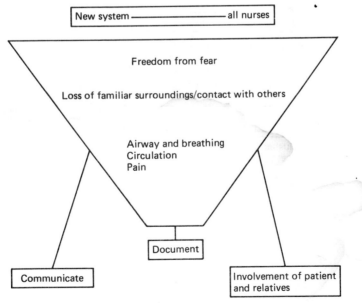

Figure 6.6 The new system incorporating the old system.

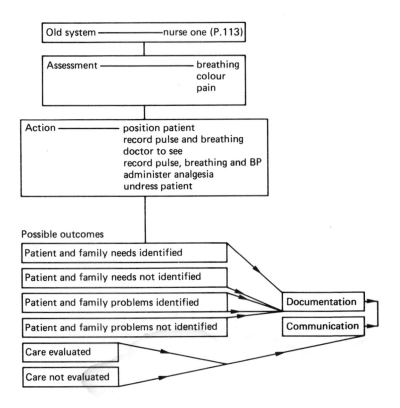

Figure 6.7 The new system versus the old system.

Versus

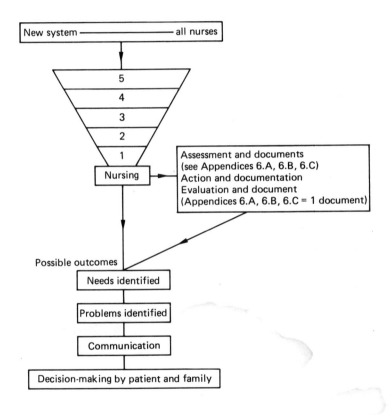

Figure 6.7 *continued.*

REFERENCES

Benner, P. (1982) 'From novice to expert,' *Am. J. Nurs.*, March, p. 402–7.

Castledine, G. (1986), cited in B. Kershaw and J. Salvage (1986) *Models for nursing* (Chichester: John Wiley & Sons).

Frought, S.G. and Trowe, A.N. (1984) *Psychosocial nursing care of the emergency patient* (Chichester: John Wiley & Sons).

Kershaw, B. and Salvage J. (1986) *Models for nursing* (Chichester: John Wiley & Sons).

Maslow, A.H. (1954) *Motivation and personality* (London: Harper and Row).

Minshull, J., Ross, K. and Turner, J. (1986) *The human needs model of nursing'*, *J. Adv. Nurs.* vol. 11, pp. 643–9.

Pearson, A. (1986) cited in B. Kershaw and J. Salvage (1986) *Models for nursing* (Chichester: John Wiley & Sons).

Roper, N., Logan, W.W. and Tierney, A. (1983) *Using a model for nursing* (Edinburgh: Churchill Livingstone).

Roper, N., Logan, W.W. and Tierney, A. (1985) *The elements of nursing* (Edinburgh: Churchill Livingstone).

Reilly, D. (1975) 'Why a conceptual framework?', *Nurs. Outlook*, vol. 23, no. 9, pp. 566–99.

Walsh, M.H. (1985) *A and E nursing: A new approach* (Heinmann).

Wright, S. (1986) *Building and using a model for nursing* (London: Edward Arnold).

FURTHER READING

Chapman, C.M. (1985) *Theory of nursing: practical application*: Lippincott Nursing Series (New York: Harper & Row).

Salvage, J. and Kershaw, B. (1990) *Models for nursing* 2 (London: Scutari Press).

Chapter 7

Nurses and nursing models: comfort or conflict?

CONTENTS

- Introduction
- What is role?
- The role of the A and E nurse
- Job satisfaction – is this related to the use of nursing models?
- Stress
- Stress, nursing process and nursing models
- The personal construct theory
- References
- Further reading

INTRODUCTION

In debates about the use of nursing models in clinical practice it is important to consider whether the discussion should include:

- Issues that may influence acceptance or rejection of them;
- The effect of other issues on the use of nursing models in clinical practice.

Three issues are to be explored in this chapter: role, job satisfaction and stress. These factors may be responsible for nurses' willingness or reluctance to examine the use of nursing models within their own areas of practice, and the reader will play an important part in the discussion that follows.

In this chapter, the reader is encouraged to address some of the problems relating to the use of nursing models. Thus, a basis is provided for exploration of nursing models within their own A and E department.

WHAT IS ROLE?

The Collins English Dictionary (1989) defines role as a specific task or function. This definition has been developed by Levinson (1959), who regards role as being made up of the thoughts and actions of an individual. He also believes that the individual's thoughts and actions are influenced by society. This concept includes social demands and 'standardizing forces'.

'Standardizing forces', in this definition, suggests that society measures and judges the individual's behaviour against established criteria.

A person's role ensures that she works within a given set of rules. These then determine her thoughts and behaviour. Pugh (1966) supports Levinson's definition. He views role as a set of expectations and behaviours associated with a given social position. This definition is connected to group interaction. The individual rarely functions in isolation. Usually she is part of a group: family, work organization. Interaction within the group helps to shape the individual's thoughts and actions. Levinson (1959), in continuing his definition, distinguishes between role and social position. Role is *related but different* to social position. Social position is a person's place within a group or organization: 'a location in social space'. Role is determined by the individual's ability to adapt her behaviour to meet the needs and rules of the group. Levinson goes on to qualify this, using the following criteria:

- Role may be connected to a person's social position. It is the result of 'structurally given demands': rules, regulations and expectations. Such demands are laid down by the group and will affect any person in any given position. It is these demands upon the individual that will provide a role, not the person's social position, although role may help establish a person's social position within the group.

Levinson identifies a difference between holding a role and occupying a social position. An individual *cannot* occupy a role (Figure 7.1).

Points for discussion:

- How does this relate to your role as an A and E nurse?
- Role is an individuals's understanding of the part she plays in a particular society. This is made up of assumptions, beliefs and ideas that particular behaviours are expected by society from the individual. This leads to the individual placing constraints upon herself. The outcome of such action is the production of a role or number of roles.

Points for discussion:

- Discuss how assumptions, beliefs and ideas may mould your work role.
- Role is a set of actions that can be matched against the individual's perception of what is 'normal'. By adopting particular actions, the individual hopes to be able to function within a specific society and be viewed was 'normal'.

Points for discussion:

- Discuss which actions by nurses may be considered 'normal' and which may not.

Many writers include all of these statements in their definition of role (Linton, 1945; Newcomb, 1950). Kincey and Kat (1984) acknowledge that the concept of role has been used in various ways by those studying psychology and sociology. Their definition of role includes the effects of group interaction upon the individual. This supports the general definitions described by Levinson (1959) and Pugh (1966). Such interaction within a group shapes and regulates the behaviour of each group member.

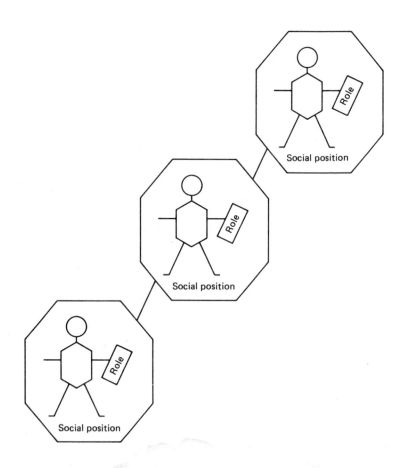

Figure 7.1 Holding a role within a social position.

Role links together an individual's perception of self and others. Perception of group members in social and work settings appears to mould the behaviour of each group member.

Points for discussion:

- How did you perceive the role of the nurse before you commenced your training?
- How may non-nurses perceive your role as a nurse?
- What is likely to influence their perception?

From the information presented so far, it can be seen that role is the result of an individual's interaction within a group. Individuals who function within group (e.g. family and work) are subjected to constraints. From such constraints the individual is led to behave in a particular way.

Role formation seems to happen within groups and is directly related to the largest group to which an individual can belong: society. The individual's role is likely to be maintained by the rules, regulations, norms and demands of any group in which they play a part. This may be the family unit, the informal work group, formal work group, or society as a whole.

Points for discussion:

- How did your role develop?
- Compare your answer with those of your colleagues.
- Describe the roles of patients and their relatives.
- How do they acquire these roles?

For relatives and patients to be given a role in A and E they have to meet certain expectations and follow certain rules.

Points for discussion:

- From where do they obtain their information about expectations and rules?

Roles also include rights and obligations (Kincey and Kat, 1984), and the individual experiences these as a result of belonging to and functioning within a particular group.

Each individual works within a specific number of roles. For example, family roles include father, mother, child, grandparent, and the roles of the nurse in A and E may include caregiver, educator, manager and health promoter.

Points for discussion:

- Describe the components that make up your role, as an A and E nurse.

Levinson's (1959) definition of role is clarified here:

- Role expectations are a set of demands and responsibilities considered normal and associated with a particular
  position;
- Role is related to the individual's understanding of what
  someone in her position is supposed to think and do;
- Role is an individual's behaviour within a given position.
  Added to this are the other parts of the individual: personality, abilities, attitudes.

Gross *et al* (1958) would include legitimate expectations;
obligations and illegitimate expectations; pressures and
stress within their definition of role.

Points for discussion:

- Discuss possible legitimate and illegitimate role expectations placed upon you, socially and at work.

Levinson (1959) views personality as playing a part in the
formation and maintenance of role. Personality affects the
way the individual adapts to a particular environment.
Their values, self identity and goals will help to mould their
role. By adapting to the environment, the individual is also
attempting to make sense of her surroundings and her place
within it. The resultant role provides the individual with
the means of creating balance within a given environment.
Change and conflict arising from the individual's need for
conformity and autonomy can be addressed within the
security of a definite role.

Points for discussion:

- Consider your role as an A and E nurse. How is it shaped
  by your personality?
- Compare your personality to that of your colleagues. How
  is their role affected by their/your personality?

Conflict may occur within working groups, when individuals have differing role expectations (Kincey and Kat, 1984).
Role conflict may follow as the individual is subjected to
incompatible role expectations.

Krech *et al* (1962) state that role conflict is produced when
an individual holds a position in two or more differing social

systems. For example, the conflict arising from combining social and work roles within an individual.

Thibaut and Kelly (1961) describe intrapersonal role conflict and Simmel (1955) describes role incompatibility. All have their roots in the differences arising from individual and group expectations.

Points for discussion:

- Have you experienced role conflict?
- What was responsible for this role conflict?

Role set is the group to which the individual belongs. Group members hold similar roles to her. Role conflict may occur when the individual's expectations differ from those of her role set.

Points for discussion:

- Describe your role set.
- How may the expectations of your role set produce role conflict within you?

Hare (1962) states that role collision may occur when two individuals hold roles that overlap. For example, nurses of the same grade in A and E who come into contact with and provide care for a patient within the department

Points for discussion:

- How may this produce role collision or conflict?

Levinson (1959) describes role demands. These are produced from particular roles. The role may be as the result of required behaviour within the organization. For example, in nursing there is the Code of Professional Conduct, standards and policies all of which influence role development. Roles are also moulded by philosophies, personal and organizational. Such philosophy may be explicit or implicit (see Chapter 2).

Points for discussion:

- Are the demands placed upon you the result of explicit, clear statements or implicit ideas?

- Where do rules and expectations come from?
- Describe how informal and formal groups may affect your work role.

Example of role conflict in A and E

The nurse encourages the relatives to be involved in the care of the patient, and, by doing this, she is fulfilling part of her role.

However, she then finds that by ensuring that involvement is encouraged, the patient and family cannot agree on the type of care the patient requires at home. Thus, in fulfilling a part of her role the nurse has created/encouraged conflict within the patient and family. This may produce problems for the nurse as she perceives that her actions have not met laid down expectations, that of caregiver, and role conflict may occur.

Points for discussion:

- Discuss how role conflict may be overcome in this situation.
- How may role conflict be overcome in other situations?

Weber (1947) provides a theory of bureaucracy that incorporates the notion of role. The bureaucratic organization is seen as a gigantic structure. Boundaries for behaviour are determined and there is strict adherence to them. Every individual has a clearly defined role and remains within the boundaries of this role. This ensures that creativity and change are restricted. Formation and maintenance of individual roles in the organization within such constraints serves to reinforce the needs and overall function of the organization.

Within the bureaucratic society there is adherence to a principle of discipline. This ensures that each member of the organization remains within the confines of her role and performs jobs as efficiently as possible. The whole system relies upon intelligent decision-making and obedience of the individuals. Emotion cannot be accepted within this structure. It is viewed as hindering efficiency.

Implicit in the theory of bureaucracy are the concepts of conformity (acceptance of group norms) and status seeking (the desire to advance oneself by the acquisition of technical competence).

Points for discussion:

• How does the bureaucratic organization differ from the A and E organization?
• How may the bureaucratic organization affect the use of nursing models in practice?

THE ROLE OF THE A AND E NURSE

In defining the role of the A and E nurse, the following points should be considered.

• Describe your *nursing* role.
• How do your colleagues define their role?
• If asked to qualify the role of the nurse in A and E, what sort of information would you present?
• How has the role of the A and E nurse changed over the last 10 years?

JOB SATISFACTION – IS THIS RELATED TO THE USE OF NURSING MODELS?

Is there a link between the acceptance or rejection of nursing models and job satisfaction? Before this question can be answered some theories of job satisfaction will be explored. As theories are introduced they will be related to nursing in A and E and to the use of nursing models.

The first theory of job satisfaction is the **motivation-hygiene theory** (Herzberg *et al*, 1959). This is based upon analysis of experiences and feelings relating to the jobs of 200 engineers and accountants in nine companies. They were asked to describe their job experiences and to group these into exceptionally good and bad experiences. They were also asked to describe how their feelings were influenced by these experiences. Favourable job attitudes were found to be related to the content of the job. These were considered intrinsic and were classed as *motivators*, associated with achievement, recognition, the work itself, responsibilities and advancements. Unfavourable job attitudes were associated with environmental factors (i.e. events extrinsic to the person) and were called *hygiene factors*. They were linked to company policy, administration, supervision, working conditions, fellow workers and personal life.

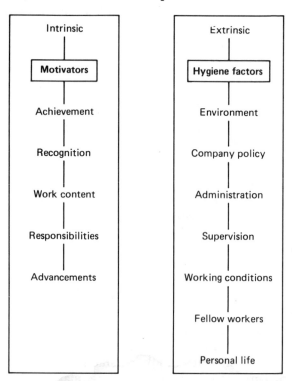

It can be concluded from this theory that motivators were more likely to produce job satisfaction. They were necessary for meeting self esteem and self actualization needs (Maslow, 1943).

Points for discussion

- What are the motivators in your job?
- Describe how motivators produce job satisfaction.

Hygiene factors, producing job dissatisfaction, were related to the inability of the person to meet needs due to outside influences. A concept of two different dimensions of job satisfaction was therefore created.

Points for discussion:

- Consider which needs, if not met, could produce job dissatisfaction for you.
- Are the needs of the nurse related to her ability to successfully practise particular skills?
- Would a nursing model highlight the skills of nurses in A and E?

There was support for this theory (Whitsett and Winslow, 1967) and criticism (House and Wigdor, 1967; Griffin and Bateman, 1986). Lack of support was due to the belief that biased results had been obtained by Herzberg and his colleagues. Further work has highlighted that generally individuals tend to view good experiences as being caused by their own actions and bad experiences as the result of events outside of them. However, Herzberg *et al's* work did draw attention to the importance of achievement and work content as factors contributing to job satisfaction.

Points for discussion:

- Describe your job.
- With reference to the above, list that which promotes job satisfaction and that which promotes job dissatisfaction.

The next theory, the **need gratification theory**, was put forward by Wolf (1970). It is related to the ability of an individual to meet her needs (Maslow, 1943). The need gratification theory states that job satisfaction will be realized if needs are met. Likewise, job dissatisfaction will result if needs are not met.

Points for discussion:

- Relate this theory to your job in A and E.
- With reference to this theory, describe the use of any model of nursing and its possible effects upon you.

Wolf's theory has been criticized, and subsequent testing has shown that needs cannot be measured accurately. Consequently, it has been considered impossible to determine whether such needs are met adequately either through work or by other means (Salancik and Pfeffer, 1977). However, this theory does reflect the importance of attitude and motive awareness in relation to work, job satisfaction and research techniques.

Points for discussion:

- Describe your needs in relation to your job.
- Organize these in order of priority.
- Give your definition of job satisfaction.
- Compare your definition with those of your colleagues.

Vroom (1964) described **the needs fulfilment theory**. In this theory, outcomes (pay and status) are measured by an individual against those outcomes received by others who are perceived to be equal. For example, a G grade nurse may expect to get the same outcomes (skills obtained as a result of post-registration education) as another G grade nurse. Acquisition of such skills may then lead to increased expectations for financial rewards. G grade nurses may measure their financial outcomes against those of social workers, a perceived equal group.

In this way, individuals assess their positions in the organization and society. The individual's value of self should be reflected in the amount of outcomes received. Should outcomes fall short of the individual's measurements, job dissatisfaction will result. Should a G grade nurse not receive education and financial rewards as she believes she should, job dissatisfaction may result. Again, attitudes to self, others, work and rewards play a large part in this theory.

Points for discussion:

- Do you measure your outcomes (pay, grading, work content) against other 'equal' individuals?
- Who are these individuals?

Hulin (1966) and Form and Geshwender (1962) provide evidence that a social group can act as a reference point for the individual. From this group the individual looks for guidance for her attitudes. The social group can be referred to as the **social reference group** and may determine application of the needs fulfilment theory.

Points for discussion:

- Can you identify a social reference group with your department?
- How can a social reference group be used to introduce a model of nursing into an A and E department?

Korman (1971) also identifies social reference groups and relates them to job satisfaction. This is supported by Cartright and Zander (1960). Blood and Hulin (1967) found blue collar workers more susceptible to social group pressure within the work environment.

The Michigan model of life satisfaction views job satisfaction as being part of the individual's past experiences. It suggests that comparisons with others and past life experiences are the main predictors of the **goal achievement gap**. This is the distance between what is wanted by the individual and what is achieved. This can then help predict job satisfaction. This model has been supported by Michalos (1980) and Locke (1976).

Points for discussion:

- How can this theory be related to the acceptance or rejection of nursing models?

As mentioned earlier, Salancik and Pfeffer (1977) criticized all need satisfaction models on the ground that further tests do not produce the same results. They put forward **the social information processing model**, arguing that job satisfaction is a socially constructed interpretation of the work situation. This theory is derived from observations of workers in various work environments.

Points for discussion:

- Using this theory, describe how nurses may perceive nursing models.

This theory is supported by Thomas and Griffin (1983). They reviewed 10 studies, most of which were conducted in laboratories. They found that the social setting of work and the worker's perceived place within that organization was derived by comparing self with others and affected the amount of job satisfaction experienced.

The job description index (Smith *et al*, 1969) states that job satisfaction is measured by examining an individual's present job: work content, pay, opportunities for promotion, supervision and colleagues.

Points for discussion:

• How may the factors described by Smith *et al* affect your perception of nursing model use in A and E?

The link between high levels of stress and job dissatisfaction has been the basis of work done by Power and Sharp (1988). They were particularly interested in the relationship between nursing stress, job satisfaction and nursing specialities. Gray-Toft and Anderson (1981) produced the **nursing stress scale**. With this, they compared the stress experienced in different types of nursing environments. They identified workload, feeling inadequately prepared to meet the emotional needs of patients and their families, and death and dying as sources of stress. These findings correspond with those of Power and Sharp (1988), Mackay (1988) and Dewe (1987).

Points for discussion:

• Describe how use of a nursing model may help the nurse overcome some of these feelings.
• How may a nursing model increase the nurse's feelings of inadequacy?

Overall, sources of job satisfaction for nurses seem to be job security, good atmosphere at work, being allowed to use skills, opportunities for further training and promotion, support of colleagues and supervisors and being able to monitor and meet patients' emotional needs.

The sources of job dissatisfaction are closely related to the value a nurse places on personal skills, the specialty in which she works and her perceived place within the work organization.

Points for discussion:

- From your understanding of the use of nursing models, which of the above factors may be associated with the use of nursing models?
- Which may not?

STRESS

Many of the modern definitions of stress are related to physiological, homeostatic models (Cooper, 1981). Cooper cites work by Lazarus (1976) who defines human stress as 'a broad class of problems differentiated from other problem areas because it deals with any demand which taxes the system, whatever it is, a physiological system, a social system, or a psychological system, and the response of that system'.

With reference to this definition, the response of an individual depends upon conscious or unconscious evaluation of a dangerous or challenging event. Stress can therefore be a 'misfit' between the individual and the environment (Cooper, 1981). The person–environment model (Cooper, 1981) is supported by Caplan (1964) and Kahn (1970)

Points for discussion:

- Which factors within your work environment create stress?

Cox (1986) describes a stimulus-based definition of stress. This takes into account disturbing and disruptive environments, and is based upon the engineering model. Cox's model of stress recognizes external stressors and their possible effects upon the individual.

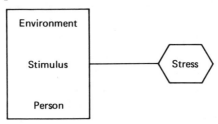

Cox supports his model by using Hooke's Law of Elasticity.

This law describes stress as being the result of a load placing demands upon a metal. Too heavy a load results in strain and deformation. If the strain produced by a given amount of stress falls within the 'elastic limit' of the material, the material will return to its normal shape once the stress is removed. Should the stress pass beyond the 'elastic limit' then permanent damage to the material will result.

Cox (1986) suggests that just as a material will have a certain resistance to stress, so have humans. Individuals can accept a certain amount of stress and deal with it on a physiological and psychological basis. Once their limit is exceeded, then some sort of damage will occur. Situations where stress may be experienced include extremes of sensory stimulation, physical hard work, insufficient work and boredom.

Weitz (1970) describes rapid information processing, an unpleasant environment, disequilibrium within the individual, isolation, group pressure and frustration as likely causes of stress.

Lazarus (1976) includes any perceived threat as a prerequisite to stress. The causes of stress are 'multifactorial and interactive' (Cooper, 1981; Carruthers, 1976). The ability to cope will depend upon the individual's perception of the threat or challenge and her physical and psychological health (Cooper, 1981).

Stress can be viewed as a physiological adaptation to demands placed upon the body. Such adaptation has been described as **the general adaptation syndrome** and is made up of three phases: reaction, resistance, exhaustion (Selye, 1976). Physiologically, the body has to maintain a perfect internal balance: homoeostasis. In the past, the stress response has been necessary to maintain homoeostasis following perceived or actual danger: the 'fight or flight' response.

In modern life, the individual may not come up against a life or death situation, but modern stressors are still able to produce a physiological reaction as the individual reacts to and attempts to adapt to daily living. Stressors stimulate the sympathetic nervous system and the release of adrenal catecholamines from the adrenal medulla. For most daily events this results in the individual becoming alert and dealing with stimuli. Should events be perceived as threatening to the individual, the second phase of the general adaptation syndrome will be reached as the individual attempts to resist the stressor. This may involve specific physiological responses such as insomnia, loss of appetite or over eating, and muscular tension.

When the individual is no longer able to maintain adaptation to the situation, the third phase is reached. This may culminate in general exhaustion or abnormal changes in the body's physiology. For example, a gastric ulcer or hypertension. Selye's description of the general adaptation syndrome can be defined as a **stress response**. In modern society, the requirement to defend the body from injury by fight or flight is rarely necessary. Stimuli that produce the stress reaction within the body in industrial society may result from frustration or anger. Situations which promote a perceived loss of control for the individual may be responsible for the body's physiological response as defined by the general adaptation syndrome. Montague (1980) describes the modern stress reaction as **maladaption**.

Points for discussion:

• How would you define stress?
• What situations in A and E are likely to lead you to experience stress?
• How would you recognize your physiological responses to stress?

Welford (1973) considers stress to be beneficial to the body. Man has evolved to function under a certain amount of stress. Inability of the body's internal environment to respond correctly is considered the root of the problem leading to possible maladaption.

Points for discussion:

• Is the ability to experience stress learnt?
• How does stress experienced at work influence your behaviour?

Cox and Mackay (1976) view stress within a transactional model. Stress is the result of an imbalance within the individual as demands are placed upon her and an inability to cope is perceived by the individual. Coping is seen as psychological 'cognitive and behavioural strategies' as well as physiological. Should normal coping be insufficient, then stress occurs resulting in abnormal physiological and psychological responses. Prolonged abnormal responses as a result of stress are liable to produce damage to the body. Cox and Mackay acknowledge that stress in individuals can be difficult to predict as each individual reacts differently to a given stimulus. This is supported by Clark and Montague (1980). Reactions to stimuli can be related to past experiences of the individual, interpretation of the stimuli and specific coping mechanisms. Coping (Clark, 1984) is a response by an individual that is then evaluated. Evaluation results in continuance or adaptation of the response by the individual.

The ability to cope with a demand leads to positive feelings of self esteem, but inability to cope leads to stress. Stress then leads to attempts at further adaptation as described by Selye (1976).

Points for discussion:

• Lack of time, insufficient communication skills and reduced autonomy have all been described as responsible for stress in nurses. Discuss these in relation to yourself and your colleagues.

Sources of work stress

Sources of work stress (Cooper, 1981) have been defined in the following ways.

The job

Jobs that result in too much or not enough work, difficult deadlines and insufficient time can give rise to stress in the individual. This can also be the case with jobs in which there are lengthy journey times taken to get to work, use of public transport and coping with traffic. Stress can be caused by a change in job and making mistakes. Sofer (1970) adds decision-making to this.

Points for discussion:

- Describe which parts of your job may encourage a stress reaction.

Working conditions

Unpleasant working conditions may be responsible for poor mental health. Such working conditions may involve the individual expending a lot of physical energy at work while, at the same time, having to meet deadlines. Repetitive work can also increase stress.

Points for discussion:

- Describe your working conditions.

Work overload

This can be divided into quantitative and qualititative overload. Quantitative is when the individual has 'too much to do' and qualititative is when the work is 'too difficult to do'.

French and Caplan (1973) have found that job dissatisfaction, job tension, low self esteem, threat, high cholesterol levels, increased heart rate, skin resistance and smoking are all produced by quantitative and qualititative work loads. This is qualified by Cooper who does not view these in isolation to the individual's personality and coping mechanisms.

Points for discussion:

- Consider what makes up your workload over one shift.
- Which parts of your workload could be responsible for stress?

Role ambiguity

This is related to the individual having insufficient information about her work role. In other words, what is expected of the individual by management and colleagues is not made clear. Role ambiguity can be responsible for job dissatisfaction, low self esteem and confidence. These can be directly related to stress (Kahn *et al*, 1964; French and Caplan, 1970). Stress as a result of role ambiguity has also be found to be responsible for mood swings, low motivation to work and intention to leave the job.

Points for discussion:

- Can you identify ambiguity within your own role?
- Could it be responsible for job dissatisfaction and stress as described above?

Role conflict

This results from conflicting job demands and a clash of expectations between the individual, colleagues and management. This may lead to the behaviour of the individual being different to that of others working within similar roles. Role conflict has been held responsible for job dissatisfaction and stress. This is increased when the individual perceives those shaping her role as powerful and authoritarian.

Points for discussion:

- How could you identify role conflict within yourself?

Responsibility

This may be responsibility for people, machines or budgets. Responsibility for others includes time spent in interaction. Trying to meet deadlines for tasks and having insufficient time to complete work are associated with failure of personal responsibility and may result in stress.

Points for discussion:

- What are your responsibilities?
- How could they contribute to stress?

Relationships at work

Positive relationships are necessary if an individual's physical and psychological health are to be maintained. Distrust of colleagues has been seen to result in high role ambiguity, loss of communication network, low job satisfaction and individual loss of self esteem (Kahn *et al*, 1964; French and Caplan, 1970).

Points for discussion:

• Consider other ways in which poor work relationships may produce stress.

Career development pressure

This can be related to promotion. There may be insufficient opportunities resulting in frustration for the individual. Alternatively, individuals may be given jobs that require more of them than they think they are able to give.

Points for discussion:

• Consider your own career development – has success or failure contributed to stress?

Commitments outside work

These may include responsibilities to family and friends. Managing time and commitments relating to work and family may lead to stress within the individual.

Points for discussion:

• How do the above factors influence your perception of the use of nursing models in nursing practice?

STRESS, NURSING PROCESS AND NURSING MODELS

According to Tschudin (1985), patients and their suffering are not the only factors inducing stress in nurses. The hospital system also contributes. She divides stress related factors into four broad categories: the introduction of the nursing process, the increase of high technology, use of equipment for patient care and demands placed on nurses as patients become more aware of treatment and care and request information about this. The nursing process has been seen as too time consuming, another name for what nurses have always done.

Morgan (1983) states that the nursing process 'encourages

greater intimacy between nurses and patients in effectively stripping away the defence mechanisms which nurses were able to use in the days when patients were illnesses and not people'.

Points for discussion:

- How does this relate to work stress as described by Cooper (1981)?
- In which ways do you consider the nursing process could be responsible for stress experienced by nurses?

Use of the nursing process requires the nurse to take more responsibility for the care of the patient (Tschudin, 1985; Faulkner, 1985). This has led to the suggestion that nurses should devise philosophies that make responsibilities associated with patient care explicit (Bamber, 1988).

Points for discussion:

- With reference to Cooper (1981), how could increasing the nurse's responsibility for the care of the patient increase stress?
- From your experience of providing care for patients, does an increase in responsibility for care giving promote stress?

The nursing process may be related to changing philosophies in nursing and the spirit of enquiry that has developed (Long, 1981). Role ambiguity and conflict may have resulted during the introduction of the nursing process.

Points for discussion:

- Are you aware of the ways in which the nursing process was introduced?
- If *yes*, describe the involvement of clinical nurses.
- Describe the effects upon nurses providing care for patients.
- If *no*, ask colleagues to give their impressions of its introduction.

The introduction of the nursing process has been viewed as emotionally demanding upon nurses (Tschudin, 1985). Many nurses confronted by the nursing process had been trained using the framework of the medical model. Many of them may have felt insufficiently prepared to work within a new framework of care delivery.

Points for discussion:

- What long-term effects has this had on the nursing profession?
- What effects do you believe that the nursing process and nursing models have/would have upon you as a nurse working in A and E?
- How do you feel about the use of nursing models in A and E and why?

Nursing models are now used in conjunction with the nursing process. Nurses work within multidisciplinary teams whose members may use other care/treatment frameworks. For example, doctors use the medical model.

Points for discussion:

- Discuss the similarities and differences between the medical model and one nursing model.
- Can nursing models be utilized appropriately within a multidisciplinary team?

THE PERSONAL CONSTRUCT THEORY

People are constantly trying to make sense of the world around them. From this observation **the personal construct theory** has developed (Kelly, 1955).

An individual may view the world differently to others; they construe events (Kelly, 1955). According to the Collins English Dictionary (1989) to construe is to interpret, deduce. An individual, therefore, interprets what she is experiencing in a unique way. Such interpretation may be very different to other individual's interpretation of the same events. The result of construing events is to produce a construct; a mental picture of what experienced events mean to the individual. A construct helps the individual make sense of her environment and ensures the individual is able to differentiate between people and events. The personal construct theory sees reality as being composed of an infinite number of

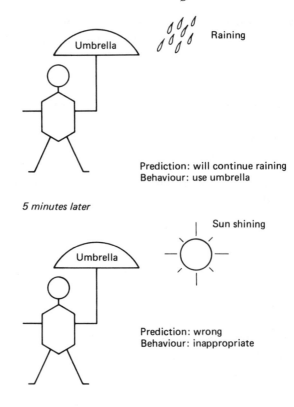

Figure 7.2   Predicting events determines behaviour.

constructs, and that reality can be constructed in any way by the individual. In trying to make sense of the world in which they find themselves, individuals have to predict what will happen (Skevington, 1984). The individual is then able to behave in a particular way. To predict events accurately the individual relies upon past experiences and relevant knowledge. These predictions are then tested (Figure 7.2).

Prediction of events by the individual allows her to decide on appropriate behaviour. If predictions turn out to be wrong, the individual may become distressed and attempt to alter her behaviour. Further attempts to understand and make predictions aim to give the individual power over future events that may be similar to those just experienced.

Positive feedback, from everything within the environment, is necessary if the individual is to maintain control over reality. Feedback from the environment enables the individual to evaluate her construction of reality, prediction of events and resultant behaviour.

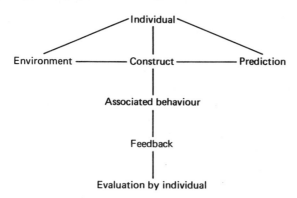

Points for discussion:

- Within a group, discuss individual interpretations of work situations.
- Discuss the outcomes of these situations and their effects upon individuals.

At work, cognitive construction and associated predictions by an individual should lead to appropriate behaviour. Positive feedback from colleagues and seniors should then promote feelings of security and control within the individual. A constantly changing work environment may prompt the individual to modify her construction of the environment, and inability to predict events and determine behaviour may produce feelings of insecurity.

Nurses need to be able to appreciate how they make sense of the world both inside and outside nursing. As has already been stated, anxiety and distress may result if an individual cannot predict events. This is especially so in nursing where new ideas and change affect the working environment. Until the nurse finds new constructs to deal with the situation the anxiety and distress will continue. Once new constructs are acquired and the construct system developed, anxiety and distress should be reduced (Skevington, 1984).

Points for discussion:

- Many changes are occurring in nursing at the moment. How would you apply the personal construct theory to individuals involved in these changes?
- Introduction of a nursing model may produce positive and negative feelings within nurses. How would you apply the personal construct theory to such feelings experienced by nurses?

Prediction of changes in a negative direction by the individual may result in inability to learn and adapt. Development of the construct system will depend upon the individual being able to establish new predictions relating to events. Should old strategies be kept then the construct system cannot be modified and developed. Old ways of dealing with the environment may need to be reviewed and new ways of constructing the world considered.

Points for discussion:

- Relate this to the use of nursing process and nursing models in A and E.
- In your experience, do nurses attempt to retain established practices when faced with the introduction of a nursing model?
- If established practices are retained, will stress result?
- How would you recognize such stress?
- What are the reasons for the acceptance or rejection of nursing models?
- Where do your colleagues stand on this issue – comfort or conflict?

REFERENCES

Bamber, M. (1988) *'Slant on stress'*, *Nursing Times*, March 16, vol. 84, no. 11, pp. 61–3.
Blood, M.R. and Hulin, C.L. (1967) *'Alienation, environmental charac- teristics and worker responses'*, *J. Appl. Psych.*, vol. 51, pp. 284–90.
Caplan, G. (1964). *Principles of preventive psychiatry* (New York: Tavistock).
Carruthers, M.E. (1976) *'Risk factor control'*, (paper presented at the conference 'Stresses of the air traffic control officer', Manchester)

cited in P.B. Warr (Ed.) (2nd ed.) (1981) *Psychology at work* (Harmondsworth: Penguin).

Cartright, D. and Zander, A. (1960) *Group dynamics: research theory* (2nd ed.) (Illinois: Peterson).

Clark, M. and Montague, S. (1980) 'Introduction', *Nursing*, vol. 1, no. 10, pp. 418–21.

Clark, M. (1984) 'Stress and coping: constructs for nurses', *J. Adv. Nurs.*, vol. 9, pp. 3–13.

Collins English Dictionary (1989) (London: Collins).

Cooper, C. (1981) '*Work stress*', in P.B. Warr (Ed.) (2nd ed.) (1981) *Psychology at work* (Harmondsworth: Penguin).

Cox, T. (1986) *Stress* (London: Macmillan Press Limited).

Cox, T. and Mackay, C.J. (1976) 'A psychological model of occupational stress', (A paper presented to the Medical Research Council meeting 'Mental Health in Industry', November, London) cited in T. Cox (1986) *Stress* (London: Macmillan Press Limited).

Dewe, P.J. (1987) 'Identifying the causes of nurses stress: a survey of New Zealand nurses', *Work and Stress*, vol. 1, pp. 15–24.

Faulkner, A. (1985) *Nursing: a creative approach* (London: Bailliere Tindall).

Form, W.H. and Geshwender, J.A. (1962) 'Social reference basis of job satisfaction: the case of manual workers', *Am. Sociol. Revi.*, vol. 27, pp. 228–36.

French, J.R.P. and Caplan, R.D. (1970) 'Psychosocial factors in coronary heart disease', *Indust. Med.*, vol. 39, pp. 383–97.

French, J.R.P. and Caplan, R.D. (1973) 'Organizational stress and individual strain', in P.B. Warr (1981) *Psychology at work* (Harmondsworth: Penguin).

Griffin, R.W. and Bateman, T.S. (1986) 'Job satisfaction and organisational commitment', in M. Argyle (1989) *The social psychology of work* (London: Penguin).

Gray–Toft, P. and Anderson, J.G. (1981) 'Stress among hospital staff: its causes and effects', *Soc. Sci. Med.* vol. 15A, pp. 639–47.

Gross, N. Mason, W.S. and McEachern, A.W. (1958) *Explorations in role analysis* (Chichester: Wiley).

Hare, A.P. (1962) *Handbook of small group research* (New York: Free Press of Glencoe).

Herzberg, F., Mauser, B. and Snyderman, B. (1959) *The motivation to work* (Chichester: Wiley).

House, R.J. and Wigdor, L.A. (1967) 'Herzberg's dual factor theory of job satisfaction and motivation: a review of the evidence and the criticism', *Pers. Psych.*, vol. 20, pp. 369–89.

Hulin, C.L. (1966) 'Effects of community characteristics on measurements of job satisfaction', *J. Appl. Psych.*, vol. 50, pp. 185–92.

Kahn, R.L. (1970) 'Some propositions toward a researchable conceptualization of stress', in P.B. Warr (1981) *Psychology at work* (Harmondsworth: Penguin).

Kahn, R.L., Wolfe, D.M., Quinn, R.P., Snoek, J.E. and Rosenthal, R.A.

(1964) *Organisational stress: studies in role conflict and ambiguity* (New York: Wiley).

Kelly, G.A. (1955) *The psychology of personal constructs* (New York: Norton Press).

Kincey, J. and Kat, B. (1984) 'How can nurses use social psychology to study themselves and their roles?', in S. Skevington (1984) *Understanding nurses: the social psychology of nursing* (New York: John Wiley and Sons Limited).

Korman, A. (1971) *Industrial and organisational psychology* (New Jersey: Prentice Hall).

Krech, D., Crutchfield, R. S. and Ballachey, E. L. (1962) *Individual in society* (New York: McGraw Hill).

Lazarus, R. S. (1971) 'The concepts of stress and disease,' *Social Stress and Disease*, vol. 1, pp. 53–60.

Lazarus, R. S. (1976) *Patterns of adjustment* (New York: McGraw Hill).

Levinson, D. J. (1959) 'Role, personality and social structure in the organizational setting', *J. Abn. Soc. Psych.*, vol. 58, pp. 170–80.

Linton, R. (1945) *The cultural background of personality* (New York: Appleton-Century).

Locke, E. A. (1976) 'The nature and causes of job satisfaction', in T. Cox (1986) *Stress* (London: Macmillan Press Limited).

Long, R. (1981) *Systematic nursing care* (London: Faber and Faber).

Mackay, L. (1988) 'Career Women', *Nursing Times*, vol. 84, no. 10, pp. 42–44.

Maslow, A. H. (1943) 'A theory of human motivation', *Psych. Rev.*, vol. 50, pp. 370–96.

Michalos, A. C. (1980) 'Satisfaction and happiness', *Social Indicators Research*, vol. 8, pp. 385–422.

Montague, S. (1980) 'The physiological basis of the stress reaction', *Nursing*, vol. 10, February, pp. 422–25.

Morgan, M. (1983) 'Report of the Peterborough RCN centre meeting', *Nursing Times*, vol. 79, no. 48, p. 21.

Newcomb, T. M. (1950) *Social psychology* (New York: Dryden).

Power, K. G. and Sharpe, G. R. (1988) 'A comparison of sources of nursing stress and job satisfaction among mental handicap and hospice nursing staff', *J. Adv. Nurs.*, vol. 13, pp. 726–32.

Pugh, D. (1966) 'Role activation conflict: a study of industrial inspection', *Am. Sociol. Rev.*, vol. 31, pp. 835–42.

Salancik, G. R. and Pfeffer, J. (1977) 'An examination of the need satisfaction model of job attitudes', *Administrative Science Quarterly*, vol. 23, pp. 224–53.

Selye, H. (1976) *The stress of life* (New York: McGraw Hill).

Simmel, G. (1955) *Conflict and the web of group affiliations* (New York: Free Press of Glencoe).

Skevington, S. (1984) *Understanding nurses: the social psychology of nursing* (New York: John Wiley and Sons Limited).

Smith, P. C., Kendall, L. M. and Hulin, C. L. (1969) *The management of satisfaction in work and retirement* (Chicago: Rand McNally).

Sofer, C. (1970) *Men in mid career* (Cambridge: Cambridge University Press).

Thibaut, J.W. and Kelley, H.H. (1961) *The social psychology of groups* (New York: John Wiley & Sons).

Tschudin, V. (1985) 'Too much pressure', *Nursing Times*, September 11, vol. 81, no. 37, pp. 30–1.

Thomas, J. and Griffin, R. (1983) 'The social information processing model of task design: a review of the literature', *Academy of Management Review*, vol. 8, pp. 672–82.

United Kingdom Central Council for Nursing, Midwifery and Health Visiting (1984) *Code of Professional Conduct for the Nurse, Midwife and Health Visitor* (2nd edn), November (London).

Warr, P. B. (Ed.) (1981) *Psychology at work* (2nd ed.) (Harmondsworth: Penguin).

Weber, M. (1947) *'The theory of social and economic organisation'* (OUP), cited in G. Salaman and K. Thompson (1982) *People and organisations* (London: Longman for Open University Press).

Welford, A. T. (1973) 'Stress and performance', *Ergonomics* vol. 16, pp. 567–80.

Weitz, J. (1970) 'Psychological research needs on the problems of human stress', cited in T. Cox (1986) *Stress* (London: Macmillan Press Limited).

Whitsett, D. A. and Winslow, E. K. (1967) 'An analysis of studies critical of the motivator-hygiene theory', *Personnel Psychology*, vol. 20, pp. 391–415.

Wolf, M. G. (1970) 'Need gratification theory: a theoretical reformulation of job satisfaction/dissatisfaction and job motivation', *J. Appl. Psych.*, vol. 54, no. 1, pp. 87–94.

Vroom, V. H. (1964) *Work and motivation* (New York: Wiley).

FURTHER READING

Argyle, M. (1989) *The social psychology of work* (London: Penguin).

Ribeaux, P. and Poppleton, S. E. (1982) *Psychology and work* (London: The Macmillan Press Limited).

Scott, D. (1970) *The psychology of work* (London: Duckworth & Company Ltd).

Chapter 8

Towards a conclusion: a final look at the nursing model debate

The aim of this book has been to examine the continuing nursing model debate, and to explore associated issues (Figures 8.1 and 8.2). It is hoped that, as a result of reading the text, the reader is better equipped to deal with these issues and is more able to evaluate these in relation to her own clinical practice.

Points for discussion:

- Which issues relating to the use of nursing models in practice concern you?
- Which concern your colleagues?

A philosophical 'journey' has been undertaken, the aim of which has been to encourage the reader to develop ideas and ask questions about the use of nursing models in A and E departments (Figure 8.3). Development of readers' ideas should open up a wider nursing model debate. It is hoped, therefore, that a foundation has been established upon which the A and E nurse can develop ideas, put them into practice and evaluate their effects upon others. Evaluation of a clinical nursing model should promote its value for all concerned.

Points for discussion:

- How would you evaluate a clinically based nursing model?
- Who would you involve in the evaluation?

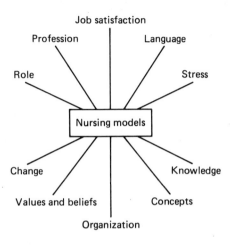

Figure 8.1 Tying up the themes.

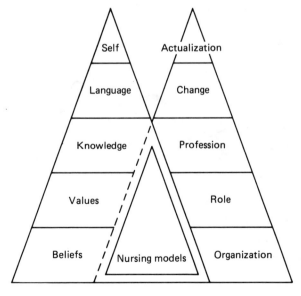

Figure 8.2 Tying up the themes.

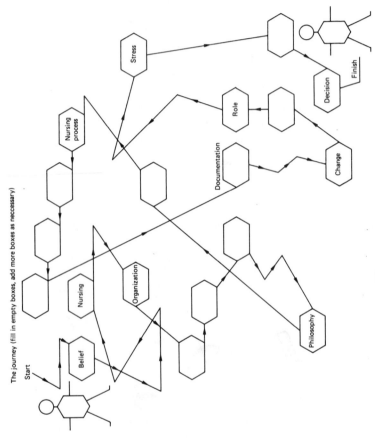

Figure 8.3 The journey.

Nursing models aim to improve patient care. Have the recipients of care been asked and by whom?

Points for discussion:

- Discuss the importance of explaining the nursing process and models to patients.
- Discuss the language used by nurses during explanation.
- What do patients want when they come into an A and E department?
- What do their families want?
- How does a nursing model fit into all of this?

Other problems and issues not addressed in this book may also become part of your nursing model debate.

Points for discussion:

- Consider the following:
  'Nurses are a problem. They are a problem for their patients, for their managers and for their government. They also cause problems for themselves' (Mackay, 1989). 'We have met an enemy and he is us' (cited in Chapman, 1983).
- How do these statements relate to the introduction of nursing models into nursing?
- How do they relate to the use of nursing models in A and E departments?
- Consider the following:
  'Most casualty work involves the categorization and early treatment of patients, rather than continuing patient care' (Hughes, 1988).
- Discuss this statement in relation to your work.
- How does a model of nursing fit into this framework of care and treatment?

Hughes (1988) goes on to state that nurses in A and E departments question patients and their families about the history of the injury. Observation of physical and psychological appearance also plays a large part in the nurse's informal assessment. The doctor may see the patient but it is the nurse who obtains much of the information through an informal assessment.

Points for discussion:

• Should the informal information gathering process be formalized through the use of a nursing model?

The role of the nurse is another important factor. Nurses should understand what they do and how they do it (Williams, 1989). How you do your job may influence your acceptance and use of a nursing model.

Points for discussion:

• Do A and E nurses understand the nature of their work?
• Is this another issue that should be explored before a nursing model is considered?

Vaughan (1989) discusses the importance of nurses *expanding* their roles and being able to offer patients a wide range of services. However, nurses should be aware of their principal role before expansion can take place.

Points for discussion:

• How does this relate to the use of a nursing model?

'Nursing practice is still based on tradition and more credence is given to 'experience' than to logical argument and rational problem solving' (Chapman, 1983). However, Williams (1989) views task orientated nursing as being responsible for destroying innovations.

Points for discussion:

• How do these statements relate to A and E nursing?
• By not utilizing nursing models, are A and E nurses aiming to protect their skills and knowledge from the public and other nurses?

'Unfortunately the possession of specialized knowledge may be jealously guarded by those who possess it, such knowledge being used to enhance power and status' (Chapman, 1983). Chapman warns that such action may backfire on nurses, 'nursing itself ceases to exist and becomes a collection of activities performed by specialist technicians'. She cites work by Thomas (1981) relating to the de-skilling of nurses, due to constant defence of special skills. De-skilling of nurses eventually results in the disappearance of nursing, because nurses fail to share their knowledge with others.

Points for discussion:

• Could use of a nursing model prevent this happening?

EPILOGUE

Points for discussion:

• Is the use of nursing models in A and E departments appropriate?

'Without a model it is impossible to practice'
(*Chalmers*, 1990)

'Far from having a positive influence on nursing practice, nursing models have placed a great burden on practitioners, and have inhibited the development of nursing expertise'
(*Kendrich*, 1990)

Points for discussion:

• What factors will influence your decision to use/not use a nursing model?

'For good or evil, man is a free creative spirit. This produces the very queer world in which we live, a world in continuous creation and therefore continuous change and insecurity'
(*Joyce Cary* 1888–1957)

Points for discussion:

• Are nursing models innovative?
• Are they part of an inevitable change process?
• Does change create insecurity for those involved in it?

'Rules and models destroy genius and art'
(*William Hazlitt* 1778–1830)

Points for discussion:

• Are nursing models responsible for restraining creativity and innovation in nursing?

The decision is yours, good luck.

REFERENCES

Chalmers, H. (1990) 'Nursing models: enhancing or inhibiting practice?,' *Nursing Standard*, December 5, vol.5, no.1, pp.34–40.

Chapman, C.M. (1983) 'The paradox of nursing,' *J. Adv. Nurs.*, vol.8, pp.269–72.

Hughes, D. (1988) 'When nurse knows best: some aspects of nurse/doctor interaction in a casualty department,' *Sociol. Health and Illness*, vol.10, no.1, pp.1–22.

Kendrich, M. (1990) 'Nursing models: enhancing or inhibiting practice?', *Nursing Standard*, December 5, vol.5, no.1, pp.34–40.

Mackay, L. (1989) *Nursing a problem* (Milton Keynes: Open University Press).

Thomas, S.P. (1981) 'The adventures of Joey in patientland: a futuristic fantasy,' *Nursing Forum*, vol.19, pp.351–57, cited in C.M. Chapman (1983) 'The paradox of nursing', *J. Adv. Nurs.*, vol.8, pp.269–72.

Vaughan, B. (1989) 'Stand up for nursing,' *Nursing Times*, July 12, vol.85, no.28, p.20.

Williams, S. (1989) 'Stand up for nursing,' *Nursing Times*, July 12, vol.85, no.28, p.20.

The A and E
nursing assessment, action and evaluation sheet
(adapted from the human needs model of nursing)

Name: *Fred Bloggs*   Presenting condition: *Chest pain*
Prefers to be called: *Fred*

Date/time of arrival in A and E: *1.1.90*   *9am.*   A and E no: *00000*

Address:

Telephone:

Date of birth: *00 00 00   62 yrs*   Religion:

Persons to be contacted:

Persons with patient in A and E: *None*

Dependants (include pets):

GP address:

Support services:

Location of property/valuables:

Location of key:

Nursing measurements recorded: Frequency:
Please refer to charts/casualty card for all recordings: *on arrival + ¼ hrly*

Temp (✓)   Pulse (✓)   Resps (✓)   BP (✓)   Others ( )   specify _____

Cardiac monitor *in situ* (✓)

The following nurse/patient problems have been identified:
① 2 3 ④ 5 6 ⑦ ⑧   please turn over

Appendix 6.A Completion of document following arrival of a
patient in A and E.

1. Airway and breathing: Position of patient (*sitting*)	**4. Pain** Area (*chest*)
Suction ( )	Type of pain (*crushing*)
Oral airway inserted ( ) Size ( )	Constant ( ) Not constant ( )
O$_2$ given (✓) L/min, % (*see cas. card*) Time commenced (*9.02*)	Analgesia given prior to arrival in A and E ( )
ET tube *in situ* ( ) Size ( )	Time ( ) By whom ( )
2. Circulation: Limbs; identify ( )	Analgesia given in A and E ( ) Time ( )
Sensation present ( ) Movement ( ) Swelling ( ) Pulses ( )	**5. Body temperature:** Patient needs cooling ( ) warming ( ) Aids used ( )
Elevated ( ) Splint applied ( )	**6. Fluid intake/output:** Oral fluids given ( )
Rings removed ( )	Nil by mouth ( )
3. Bleeding: Area ( )	IV Cannula *in situ* ( ) Site satisfactory ( )
Amount; Small ( ) Moderate ( )	IV Fluids commenced ( ) Time ( )
Large ( )	Nausea ( )
Type ( )	Vomiting ( )
Pressure applied ( )	Diarrhoea ( )
7. Loss of familiar surroundings/ contact with others:	**8. Freedom from fear** Necessity for physical examination; patient
Patient is aware where he/she is (✓) not aware ( )	aware (✓)
Relatives contacted/aware patient is in A and E ( )	relatives aware ( )
Not contacted/aware (✓) Reason (*see below* ⑦)	Reasons for medical/ nursing procedures: explanation given to
Relatives are with patient ( ) Parents present ( ) Others present ( ) specify _____	patient (✓) relatives ( ) by nursing staff (✓) medical staff ( )
Workplace contacted/aware patient is in A and E ( ) Not contacted/aware (✓) Reason (*see below* ⑦)	Advice needed by patient ( ) relatives ( ) about this injury and further employment ( )

Describe any further nursing assessment/action taken:
7. *Patient wishes his wife to be contacted ASAP – done 0905*
7. *Work place to be contacted.*

Evaluation for ① 2 3 4 5 6 7 8:
① *Airway patent – breathing satisfactory 0905*

Medication given as prescribed ( )   Time ( ) Effects of medication given _____
Patient's destination ( ) Patient aware ( ) Relatives aware ( ) Nursing sheet completed by *L. C. Sbaih*   Time (*9.05*)

Appendix 6.A continued.

The A and E
nursing assessment, action and evaluation sheet
(adapted from the human needs model of nursing)

Name: *Fred Bloggs*
Prefers to be called: *Fred*

Presenting condition: *Chest pain*

Date/time of arrival in A and E: *∅   1.1.90   9am*   A and E no: *00000*

Address:

Telephone:

Date of birth: *00 00 00   62 yrs*   Religion:

Persons to be contacted:

Persons with patient in A and E: *None   Wife arrived @ 09.15 am*

Dependants (include pets):

GP address:

Support services:

Location of property/valuables:

Location of key:

Nursing measurements recorded: Frequency:

Please refer to charts/casualty card for all recordings: *on arrival + ¼ hrly*

Temp (✓) Pulse (✓) Resps (✓) BP (✓)   Others ( ) specify _____

Cardiac monitor *in situ* (✓)

The following nurse/patient problems have been identified:
① 2   3   ④   5   ⑥   ⑦   ⑧   please turn over

Appendix 6.B Completion of document after patient is seen by doctor.

1. Airway and breathing:	4. Pain
Position of patient (*sitting*)	Area (*chest*)
Suction ( )	Type of pain (*crushing*)
Oral airway inserted ( )	Constant ( )
Size ( )	Not constant ( )
O$_2$ given (✓ L/min, % *see cas. card.*)	Analgesia given prior to
Time commenced (*0902*)	arrival in A and E ( )
ET tube *in situ* ( )	Time ( )
Size ( )	By whom ( )
2. Circulation:	Analgesia given in A and E (✓)
Limbs; identify ( )	Time (*0905*)
Sensation present ( )	5. Body temperature:
Movement ( )	Patient needs cooling ( )
Swelling ( )	warming ( )
Pulses ( )	Aids used ( )
Elevated ( )	6. Fluid intake/output:
Splint applied ( )	Oral fluids given ( )
Rings removed ( )	Nil by mouth ( )
3. Bleeding:	IV Cannula *in situ* (✓)
Area ( )	Site satisfactory (✓ *0905*)
Amount; Small ( )	IV Fluids commenced ( )
Moderate ( )	Time ( )
Large ( )	Nausea ( )
Type ( )	Vomiting ( )
Pressure applied ( )	Diarrhoea ( )

7. Loss of familiar surroundings/ contact with others:	8. Freedom from fear
Patient is aware where he/she is (✓ not aware ( )	Necessity for physical examination; patient aware (✓)
Relatives contacted/aware patient is in A and E (✓)	relatives aware (✓)
Not contacted/aware (✓) Reason (*See below* ⑦)	Reasons for medical/ nursing procedures: explanation given to
Relatives are with patient (✓) Parents present ( ) Others present ( ) specify _____	patient (✓ relatives (✓) by nursing staff (✓) medical staff (✓)
Workplace contacted/aware patient is in A and E (✓) *9.05am* Not contacted/aware (✓) Reason (*see below* ⑦)	Advice needed by patient (✓ relatives (✓) about this *visit* ~~Injury~~ and further employment (✓)

Describe any further nursing assessment/action taken:

7. *Patient wishes his wife to be ~~contacted~~ ASAP – done 0905*
7. *Work place ~~to be~~ contacted. 0905*

Evaluation for ① 2 3 ④ 5 6 ⑦ ⑧:

① *Airway patent, breathing satisfactory 0905.*
① *pt. says he is comfortable, breathing satisfactory 0910.*
④ *Still some pain but more comfortable*
      no pain 0911.
⑦ *wife wishes to remain with Fred 0915*
⑧ *Mr & Mrs Bloggs have several questions re: work.*

Medication given as prescribed ( )	Time ( )
Effects of medication given _____	

Patient's destination ( ) Patient aware ( ) Relatives aware ( )
Nursing sheet completed by _*L.C. Sbaih*_ Time (*9.05*)

Appendix 6.B continued.

**The A and E
nursing assessment, action and evaluation sheet**
(adapted from the human needs model of nursing)

Name: *Fred Bloggs*
Prefers to be called: *Fred*

Presenting condition: *Chest pain*

Date/time of arrival in A and E: *1.1.90*   *9am*   A and E no: *00000*

Address: *4, High Street*

Telephone: *00000*

Date of birth: *00 00 00   62 yrs*   ·   Religion:

Persons to be contacted:

Persons with patient in A and E: *None*   *Wife arrived @ 09.15 am*

Dependants (include pets): *None*

GP address: *Dr. Smith*

Support services: *None @ present.*

Location of property/valuables: *c̄ patient*

Location of key: *c̄ patient*

Nursing measurements recorded:

Please refer to charts/casualty card for all recordings:

Temp (✓) Pulse (✓) Resps (✓) BP (✓) Others ( ) specify _____

Cardiac monitor *in situ* (✓) *see charts × once*

Frequency:
on arrival + ¼ hrly
½ hrly

The following nurse/patient problems have been identified:
① 2 3 ④ 5 ⑥ ⑦ ⑧   please turn over

Appendix 6.C Completion of document prior to admission to CCU .

1. Airway and breathing:	**4. Pain**
Position of patient (*sitting*)	Area (*chest*)
Suction ( )	Type of pain (*crushing*)
Oral airway inserted ( )	Constant ( )
Size ( )	Not constant ( )
O_2 given (✓ L/min, % (*see cas. card*)	Analgesia given prior to
Time commenced (*0902*)	arrival in A and E ( )
ET tube *in situ* ( )	Time ( )
Size ( )	By whom ( )
2. Circulation:	Analgesia given in A and E (✓)
Limbs; identify ( )	Time (*9.05*)
Sensation present ( )	**5. Body temperature:**
Movement ( )	Patient needs cooling ( )
Swelling ( )	warming ( )
Pulses ( )	Aids used ( )
Elevated ( )	**6. Fluid intake/output:**
Splint applied ( )	Oral fluids given ( )
Rings removed ( )	Nil by mouth ( )
3. Bleeding:	IV Cannula *in situ* (✓)
Area ( )	Site satisfactory (✓ *0905*)
Amount; Small ( )	IV Fluids commenced ( )
Moderate ( )	Time ( )
Large ( )	Nausea ( )
Type ( )	Vomiting ( )
Pressure applied ( )	Diarrhoea ( )

7. Loss of familiar surroundings/ contact with others:	**8. Freedom from fear**
Patient is aware where he/she is (✓ not aware ( )	Necessity for physical examination; patient aware (✓
Relatives contacted/aware patient is in A and E (✓	relatives aware (✓
Not contacted/aware (✓	Reasons for medical/ nursing procedures:
Reason (*see below* ⑦)	explanation given to
Relatives are with patient (✓	patient (✓ relatives (✓
Parents present ( )	by nursing staff (✓
Others present ( )	medical staff (✓
specify _____	
Workplace contacted/aware patient is in A and E (✓ *9.05 am*	Advice needed by patient (✓ relatives (✓
Not contacted/aware (✓	about this *visit* ~~injury~~ and
Reason (*see below* ⑦)	further employment (✓

Describe any further nursing assessment/action taken:
7. *Patient wishes his ~~wife to be~~ contacted – done 0905*
7. *~~Workplace to be~~ contacted. 0905*

Evaluation for ① 2 3 ④ 5 6 ⑦ ⑧

① *Airway patent, breathing satisfactory 0905.*
① *pt. says he is comfortable, breathing satisfactory 0910.*
④ *Still some pain but more ~~comfortable~~*
         no pain 0911.
⑦ *wife wishes to remain with Fred 0915*
⑧ *Mr & Mrs Bloggs have several questions re: work.*

Medication given as prescribed ( )	Time ( )
Effects of medication given _____	
Patient's destination (*CCU*) Patient aware (✓ Relatives aware (✓	
Nursing sheet completed by ___ *L. C. Stair* ___ Time (*9.05*)	

To CCU 9.25 am LCS

Appendix 6.C continued.

Author Index

Subject Index